## NEW EDITION,

Completely Revised, and including adjustments and additions suggested by readers and other authorities!

# THE PENIS

by
Dr.Dick Richards MD

After years of intensive research and study, the truth is finally revealed about topics previously considered to be of the most shocking nature.

©

Published by:
BabyShoe Publications
P.O.Box 75, CT13 9RT
England

ISBN 1 874069 20 4

# Contents

Introduction

Section One:       THE PENIS MACHINE
- Chapter One:       What the Penis Is
- Chapter Two:       Semen
- Chapter Three:       The Psychology of the Penis
- Chapter Four:       Penis Technique
- Chapter Five:       The Penis Elsewhere

Section Two:       THE PENIS AROUND THE WORLD
- Chapter Six:       The Penis in Art
- Chapter Seven:       Myths and Legends
- Chapter Eight:       Penis Rituals and Phallic Worship

Section Three:       THE BROKEN PENIS
- Chapter Nine:       Diseases of the Penis
- Chapter Ten:       Sex Faults of the Penis
- Chapter Eleven:       Sexual Aids

Section Four:       THE WOMAN'S PENIS
- Chapter Twelve:       The Past and the Present
- Chapter Thirteen:       Mutual Techniques
- Chapter Fourteen:       Some Problems and Solutions

Section Five:       THE BIG PENIS
- Chapter Fifteen:       Big,... Why?
- Chapter Sixteen:       Big,... How?
- Chapter Seventeen:       The Magical Extras

Conclusion

* * * * *

# Introduction

If one were pressed to choose the one single most important object on all the Earth and in the entire history of Man upon the Earth, then, without a fragment of doubt, the final choice would have to be the human penis.

A man will, with scrupulous care, amass a financial fortune. He will create a work of art or he will invent a new surgical operation. He will conquer and lay waste an entire nation. And then he will discard all reason in his headlong pursuit of a wet T-shirt or a set of shapely shaven pudenda. He will accept the dictates of his sex drive as far as he possibly can and substitute for them where and when he cannot. However unreasonable his desires, they affect him to the very core of his existence. Knowing that his actions lack reason and logic, he will nonetheless throw away his all for the pandering of his sexual whim and the pampering of his penis.

The most spectacular revelations of history were not those of the bringers of the great new religions. No revelations of extra-terrestrial wisdom influenced as many men as deeply as the revelation of an erect penis when its foreskin is drawn back. Alexander and Napoleon led vast armies of conquest. Kublai Khan swept across half the earth to plunder Cathay. But no great commander ever gave his men the same satisfaction as they got from ejaculating into a welcoming woman. The discovery of the wheel and of the electron revolutionised the path of human events. But no discovery ever reached a man with any comparable importance as surely as did his discovery of his penis and its capacity for bringing delight.

Long ago a great wit attempted to dissuade a friend from sexual behaviour on the grounds that the position was ludicrous, the pleasure momentary and the expense damnable. But it changed nothing. Man went on being led, as it were, by the balls, as he had always been.

Since the beginning of recorded time, the penis had, figuratively as well as factually, reared its head,.. ugly or beautiful depending as much on timing as on viewpoint. When we read in the Book of Genesis of the way that woman was made from the rib of man, the rib is an acceptable and symbolic substitute for the penis. 'Ribbing' someone is poking fun,.. 'poking' is another word for having intercourse with,.. 'chewing on the spare rib' is an expression meaning fellation. All of these phrases, and others, come from the likening of the penis to a rib, just as in the Bible. It is no good counting the number of ribs of male and female. It may be a pleasure, but however often they are counted it turns out they have the same number. It is not a rib a woman lacks but a penis,.. though she does have a little replica of her own. As we shall see, much of the history of the difference between the sexes stems from this anatomical distinction.

A man may not quite recall the shape and pattern of his own arm. He may overlook the wound on his finger or the wart on his face. But, once discovered, he will never, never forget the appearance of his penis. He pays more attention to it than to anything else. He will fondle it and tend it more than anything else. He will protect it above all else. He may not know the colour of his eyes but he feels and knows every movement of his testicles. All men like to feel penis pride too, in size, shape, quality and performance. Things that erode that pride erode the man himself. The penis is all important to him. The penis leads and rules. Without it he is not the same. Nothing that affects it fails to affect him accordingly, and vice versa. It is the place where, he feels, his very *Manhood* lies. In a phrase, like it or not and recognise it or not,.. a man is his penis.

This book aims to inform, to amuse and to provoke, but throughout it is based on that hypothesis. Just one thing must be pointed out at the start. The very form and style of this book leaves me, the author, open to charges of male chauvinism. These charges would not all be really fair. Much that is written here is for the interest and guidance of men about the penis and thus, apart from Section Four, it is slanted that way. But it is also packed with data that should be invaluable to the caring woman too. Seen in that light I do not believe it will give rise to too many false impressions.

* * * * *

Written in Gwent, Wales.

#  SECTION ONE:
# THE PENIS MACHINE
**Chapter One:** What The Penis Is

Before embarking on other considerations of the penis it is necessary to give some thought to what it is, how it becomes what it is, and how it works.

To the non-technically minded and to those with no interest in physiology this can be pretty dull stuff. However, it has so much bearing on everything else there is to say that for anyone wanting seriously to read and learn, it provides the foundation. Briefly, then, we shall talk about the way the penis grows from almost nothing in the unborn child to the dominating organ of the man's body and personality. Then a short comment on its anatomy, or structure, will be followed by an explanation of its ability to erect and ejaculate, and the part it plays in sex in general and in orgasm in particular.

The penis is a sexual organ. It has no other primary purpose. To some it may look an item of beauty and adornment. To some it may represent a grotesque distorted appendage. It may look nice, feel good, smell pleasant, taste sweet. It may fascinate, horrify, delight or disgust. It can be fun to play with for its owner or his friends. Its other job, that of helping squirt unwanted urine clear of the body, may be convenient, but it is not essential. Women don't have an extending penis and they manage fairly well. So do lower animals that have no penis at all.

When all is said and done the penis is designed and constructed for sex. The job of the penis is to provide a tube passing deeply into the female body so that male germ cells, the sperms, can be deposited safely in her and have the best possible chance of making her pregnant. Everything about the penis is intended to further that aim. When it is not being sexual it is a quiet, soft little organ, tucked out of the way in a fairly safe place and causing no trouble to anyone. Sexually aroused it becomes a rigid communication duct, singularly awkward in size, shape and position for any other purpose but inseminating the female.

**The first sign of manhood**

Some women may suspect that they are pregnant within a few days of becoming so. There are not many like that. Most start to get suspicious when they miss a period, or when their breasts start to enlarge or when, at about six weeks perhaps, they start to get the first nausea and vomiting that we call morning sickness. Yet, at this stage, hidden away inside them, the tiny baby is already starting to show signs of sex.

The first visible changes are taking place which will grow into a penis. Yet the baby is still only a good deal less than half an inch long. That early start alone shows how important the penis and its sexual characteristics are.

The actual sex of the new individual is determined at the moment of conception. The mother's egg cell and the father's sperm cell each contain chemical patterns that carry the characteristics of the next generation. Whether the eyes will be blue or brown, whether the person will be tall or short, even special things like hooked noses and ways of walking are already decided by the combination of these chemical shapes, called genes. So too is decided the eventual sex of the baby to come. Looking at the minute scrap of tissue that will grow into the baby however, gives no clue to the sex. Male and female are identical, growing swiftly from a solid ball of cells to a hollow sphere of cells and eventually to a long thin object with large brain at one end and a perfectly obvious, rather tadpole-like tail at the other.

At about five weeks the tail is at its largest and after that it gradually starts to disappear. Small pieces of tissue have already formed which will be the sex glands, the ovaries for the female and the testicles for the male. Even these look the same at this stage. Now, at about six weeks, the real action begins. Between the root of the tail and the place where the umbilical cord from the mother enters the 'baby' a little lump starts to grow. It is called the genital tubercle and looks the same in both sexes.

On the side of the lump nearest the tail is a groove and on each side of it the heaped up edges of the groove grow larger. Meanwhile the tip of the tubercle gets longer and longer and after about two more weeks, through a magnifying glass it looks a bit like a tiny penis. Behind it the edges of the groove get higher and fold over to touch each other enclosing a tubular space within them. This will be the urethra, the urinary tube that runs the length of the adult penis shaft. Slowly, as the changes take place, the growing tissues start to take slightly different shapes. The development goes one way to become female and the other way to become male. Underneath the growing genital tubercle is a small cavity which becomes separated into three smaller ones,.. the anus, the vagina and the urethra in the female, and anus and urethra only in the male.

So, when the genital organs of man and woman have fully grown, the same original bits have taken the different shapes which distinguish the apparently very different outward appearances of each. We can make a list of parts which had the same origins:-

| Man | Woman |
| --- | --- |
| Testicle | Ovary |
| Bladder | Bladder |
| Penis | Clitoris |
| Scrotum | Labia Majora |

Even smaller things, the labia minora, the hymen and the vagina, the prostate gland and so on, have their counterparts in the opposite sex. We are by no means as different as we look.

**The finished product**

The final construction of the penis is a far cry from the insignificant little wart-like tubercle. Within it, as it grew, parts have become differentiated into its main sections. It is as well to discuss it learn its names and parts in detail as we shall repeatedly refer to it them in the rest of the book.

As we see it in the adult the penis has a free hanging (or, when erected, standing) portion known as the body or *shaft* of the penis and a similarly sized part buried inside the body beneath the pubic bone and called the *root*. The root of the penis is the part that is actually attached inside. The place where the body of the penis enters the body proper and becomes the root is called the *base* of the penis.

The easiest way to think of the penis is in its erect state. If you look at it, it has a skin-covered main part, the shaft. Near the tip there is a distinct *groove* all around it (called the coronal sulcus) separating the shaft from the swollen pink *head* called the glans or more commonly, the *knob*. Hanging over the knob is a loose fold of skin called the *foreskin* or prepuce. It is this skin that is removed by the operation called circumcision. So, if the penis you are looking at has been circumcised, the foreskin will be absent.

Starting at the very deepest end of the root on each side is a kind of tube full of material that looks rather like a sponge. The two tubes approach each other and become adherent to each other in the centre. Each is called a corpus cavernosum, (in English, the 'hollow body'), and is filled with blood. In the groove between and beneath the two joined tubes lies a third rather narrow tube, the corpus spongiosum (the 'spongy body'). It too, as its name tells, contains sponge-like tissue. It is the spongy body that enlarges to from the glans at its forward end. Through the centre of the spongy body is a real tube. This is the *urethra*, the tube of the penis, which opens at the glans in a hole called the *meatus* (the 'eye' of the penis). Through the urethra the urine and the semen are ejected. The upper and lower surfaces of the penis shaft are called, respectively, the dorsal and the urethral surfaces.

Between the root of the penis and the bladder is the *prostate gland*, lying around the first part of the urethra. The testicles lie in a bag of skin, the *scrotum*, beneath and behind the base of the penis. From each testicle a tube, the *vas*, (the tube that is cut in the operation of vasectomy), runs up over the front of the pubic bone where it is rather vulnerable and tender if squashed or struck, and into the body through a hole in the muscles of the abdomen. (It is through this hole very often that a rupture, or more correctly a hernia, can develop). Once inside the body, the vas, carrying the sperms, enters the prostate gland to join and open into the urethra. Almost at this point, there is a small bag attached to it, the *seminal vesicle* (the semen bag or sperm sack) in which semen is stored until wanted

Not all animals have the same sort of penis, though the basic parts are similar. For example, both dogs and cats actually have a bone in the shaft to help with the process of erection,... some feel this has been a sad omission in the case of impotent men. The shape of the penis varies pretty widely too. One of the most remarkable is that of the opossum. His glans is actually forked for about two centimetres at the tip. Curious too is the pig, whose penis is distinctly corkscrew shaped, making as much as two or three complete twists about three quarters of an inch in diameter. The penis of the bull has a pronounced longitudinal twist in the shaft. The goat and the ram each have a very thin worm-like tip to the penis up to three to four centimetres long. There are wide variations in humans too as to length, girth and the shape of the glans.

The two most essential supplies of the penis from the point of view of its job are its blood supply and nerve supply. The blood vessels are branches of larger ones inside the body, and the rate of flow of blood through them can change rapidly. This is what happens during the process of erection.

Erection is the preparation of the penis for its sexual function. The limp penis of its non-sexual phase is too soft for proper entry into the female vagina. It is necessary for it to become firmer. That it should also become longer is clearly an added advantage. In the course of as little as a few seconds in the powerfully aroused young male, the penis more than doubles in size. It juts out from the belly, a rigid, swollen member capable of considerable thrusting even into an unyielding vagina if necessary.

The stimulation that induces the process of erecting is mostly emotional or psychic though several chemical processes are also associated with this. The mind, partly as a result of what the eye sees and the ear hears, is subjected to strongly sexual thoughts. The anticipation of sexual contact, the feel of the body and especially the penis being stroked, the action of stroking the partner in return and so on, all add up to immense erotic rapture. The mind starts to involve itself in sexual ideas and the process continues. Down the spinal cord and through the other (sympathetic and parasympathetic) nerve systems, sexual stimuli reach the genitalia.

Only recently have the details of some parts of the highly complex process been discovered. Blood pumps rapidly into the penis. Affected by various chemicals including oxides of nitrogen some small valves open and others close. At the same time the veins through which blood normally leaves the penis are compressed. Blood cannot get out so easily. So it collects in the hollow and spongy bodies, filling them and swelling them to greater size. An erection starts, the base of the penis is pushed up under the pelvic bones, thus further restricting the blood from getting out. The entire organ becomes a strong bone-like structure ready for use.

During preceding hours or days, sperms produced in the testicles have passed along the vas on each side to reach the sperm sacks. The sacks then produce some liquid as do other parts of the lining and the prostate gland itself. This liquid, added to the sperms, actually forms the bulk of the semen.

While sex play is going on, the sensations from the glans, added to all the other emotional arousal, sets up a reflex action through the spinal cord. The muscles in the wall of the vas and elsewhere undergo rhythmic contractions pushing more and more contents towards the penis. Semen is squeezed out into the bottom of the urethra in readiness.

Suddenly excitement reaches a peak. This is mostly emotional, the sensation of approaching climax. During it, all feelings like discomfort, guilt, shame and other unpleasant associations are excluded from the mind. There is an overwhelming and increasing concentration on sexual involvement, thrusting, clutching, jerking, gasping, biting, and straining the hips and penis forward. The progress becomes a breathless rush until suddenly a point of no return is reached. Reflexly, and thus totally beyond control, the muscles that surround the urethra start to contract in a series of violent spasms. The semen in the urethra is subjected to a number of grasping pressures. It is forced, rushing up the urethra, to the glans to be spurted out either as drops or as a tiny jet. The mixed feelings of pleasure of the hot semen squirting up and out, the repeated contractions of the internal muscles, and the overall feelings of intense emotional excitement together constitute what is called orgasm. Other names are coming, coming off, climaxing and so on. The actual spurting out of semen is what is known as ejaculation. By some the phenomenon of orgasm is called 'coming' and the semen ejaculate is known as 'come,' or as spunk, love-juice or jism.

Immediately after coming there is, in the male, a period when further sexual excitement is difficult and unwanted if not impossible or even painful. This *refractory period* may be only a few minutes long, but is more often fifteen to twenty minutes. After that, re-arousal and further orgasms may be possible, the more so in younger age groups. The amount of ejaculate in subsequent orgasms however, is never as much as from the first orgasm one,.. in spite of a lot of talk to the contrary. Men who brag about ejaculating semen repeatedly and in great quantities are liars. Don't believe the braggarts who tell you that their semen ran in streams all over a girl from her face and chin down to her ankles. It is just wishful thinking.

## The female penis

As we saw in the embryology lesson at the start of this chapter, the woman too has a kind of penis, the *clitoris*. In miniature it is very like a penis except that it does not have a urethra up through it or a hole in its tip. It does have a tiny glans, it does have a distinct foreskin, and under the surface of the pink 'skin' which covers it, there is a body and root of spongy tissue just like the penis. When stroked and excited this enlarges in the same way and can usually be felt to become quite a firm bud or bulge under the finger tip. Also like a penis it is extremely sensitive, by far the most sensitive part of the female genitalia.

For most women it is the clitoris that produces the most pleasurable stimulation of all and is the part they rub and play with during masturbation. It is true that a woman often comes with similar thoughts, feelings and muscle movements to a man. What is not true is that she 'comes' or ejaculates, like him. Nothing comes from the clitoris. There is no hole. The only fluids she produces are the small (usually) amounts of lubrication that ooze or 'sweat' from the vagina and further up. Seldom are the amounts very large. Letters in gents magazines about making her 'juices' run in streams down her legs and so on, are almost always rubbish. Exceedingly few do this. The usual amount is seldom more than enough to moisten and lubricate the vaginal lips.

The inner surface of the foreskin of both penis and clitoris produces a thick substance of cream cheese-like consistency called *smegma*. It tends to collect under the foreskin unless regularly washed away. In addition to drying secretions, it contains cast-off skin cells and some bacteria. It can thus become dirty and infected and should be washed away with soap and water daily. However it is best not washed away too soon before intercourse as it has, for male and female alike, a scent that can produce strongly sexual arousal. Such a stimulus should never be wasted.

Another reason for washing the male smegma away regularly is that it contains a fatty substance believed capable of helping cause cancer in women. This may be why Jewish women get fewer cancers of the neck of the womb (where the penis presses during intercourse) and nuns almost never get such a condition.

\* \* \* \* \*

## Chapter Two: Semen

Semen is the final product of the male sexual organs as it is ejaculated from the penis. The word comes from the Latin word for seeds, as one of the two main constituents of semen are male reproductive cells, or sperms, more correctly called spermatozoa. To us, that knowledge seems acceptable and obvious, but that is really far from the case. Many people in the past did not know the connection. Some primitive tribes failed to grasp the association of sexual intercourse with the arrival of a new human being. Intercourse, to them, was a thing that happened often, pregnancy was a slow process of uncertain origin. The separation of the insemination process from the birth process by a time lag of nine months was enough to confuse simple minds and prevent them from grasping the relevance of one to the other.

### The sperm factory

Semen is a thick, colourless, gelatinous, non-transparent fluid similar in appearance to boiled starch. Occasionally, as a result of some disease process, it can become yellowish in colour if pus is present in it, or pinkish or even red if there is contamination by blood.

It consists of sperms and a fluid in which they live and 'swim.' The sperms are made in the testicles from cells specially set aside for the purpose from the time when the foetus is only about four to six weeks old. The sperms, each one of which carries all the characteristics of the father that can be passed on, leave the testicle and after passing along the vasa are stored in the seminal vesicles until wanted. A sperm looks rather like a microscopic tadpole. The large head-like nucleus has a long thin hair-like tail which lashes and spirals, thus propelling the 'tadpole' in the appropriate direction.

The prostate gland produces a liquid which is mixed with the sperms. So does the wall of each seminal vesicle, and some other very small (bulbo-urethral) glands nearby. The resulting mixture is the final product, semen. When ready for use only a very small percentage by volume of semen is made up of sperms. The remainder is the carrier-fluid. When the vas has been cut, as in the operation of vasectomy, no sperms can reach the storage sacks. They die and are harmlessly re-absorbed. The fluid, however, goes on being produced.

I am often asked about the effects of vasectomy. It is possible to reassure people by explaining that they will still produce semen that looks and behaves like it did before the operation. The tiny reduction in quantity as a result of the absence of sperms is scarcely noticed and anyway, as we'll soon see, it can be made up for in other ways. Vasectomised men will still have the same sex urge, the same abilities, the same power of erection. They will also ejaculate the same. The appearance, feel and taste of the semen will not alter. The sole difference will be that the semen contains no sperms. These can only be seen under a microscope,.. and who keeps a microscope in the bedroom anyway?

One of the requirements for successful sperm production is the correct temperature. Although sperms may be produced at temperatures just slightly different from that chosen by nature, if there is much variation the sperms lose their mobility and their fertility and die. This is one of the reasons why the taking of repeated hot baths can act as a partial [and unreliable] contraceptive. It is most certainly not to be depended upon, but the actual number of sperms can be reduced, as can their mobility, by repeated long soaking in hot water. The critical importance of temperature is one of the reasons why the testicles hang in the scrotum and outside the body where they are a little cooler. The testicles remain down in the scrotum in continuous breeders like man. In animals who have a particular breeding season the testicles enter the scrotum only for that season and return to the safety of the body when it is over.

**Increasing ejaculate**

As most of the semen is the secretion or product of glands, it follows that its quantity can be most easily increased by stimulating these glands. The exact mechanism of this is not known but the most powerful stimulus is sexual excitement. Throughout the waking and sleeping hours, probably under the influence of a hormonal as well as a neurological control mechanism, sperms and semen fluid are continuously produced. An increase in the frequency of intercourse certainly speeds up the process. It is the fluid rather that the sperms that increase most and most easily,.. sperms take longer. If a man ejaculates the average volume of three to five cubic centimetres and then goes on with further sexual activity, subsequent ejaculations will normally only produce about one to two cubic centimetres or less. Reckoning an ordinary teaspoon to be around 5ccs, it will be seen that rather more than half a teaspoon is about normal. Much more than this is uncommon even after long abstinence as the seminal vesicles simply have not got room for it.

The amount produced matters a lot to some people. Both he and she alike can come to regard semen as highly significant. He may take pride in his amount (rather than the quality) and she may see it as a salute to her sexual attractiveness and love-making ability to induce a large ejaculate. If it is wished to produce the maximum possible amount the best method is to abstain from ejaculation for a least two or three days, but during those days to encourage sexual thoughts frequently and to masturbate two or three times each day stopping well short of orgasm. Not only does this ensure that the reservoirs are at maximum, but by focusing the sex drive, it can pave the way for a very powerful orgasm when it comes. In a couple who enjoy watching ejaculation or in the woman who takes the ejaculate where she can actually feel it (for example, hand or mouth) this can produce a massive squirting of semen for a remarkable distance.

The distance semen will ejaculate depends partly on the amount available. More especially though, it depends on the suddenness and completeness of the contraction of the perineal muscles. If these go into violent spasm as in a really powerful orgasm it is quite possible for semen to squirt two or three yards in younger men. Perhaps twelve to fifteen inches is more of an average. Another factor is the shape of the glans and the direction in which its meatus points. In any event the distance of ejaculation is of no material significance except in those for whom it holds a visual fascination. The men (and women) who come to clinics claiming that they don't shoot as far as the men in the sex magazines don't know that clever photography and exceptional models are aided by liberal amounts of flour and water mix. A girl's face spattered with a tablespoonful of mix and then photographed as a penis ejaculates over it yields a photograph that can confuse viewers into imagining that the model really did produce so much semen shot over such a long distance. Half a teaspoon for several inches is what most men can manage most of the time.

**Things to come**

During each ejaculation the semen varies considerably between the different phases. This has been tested by the technique of masturbation onto a swiftly moving belt of nonabsorbent paper. The ejaculate lands in separate droplets which can be quickly and separately analysed. This has shown that during sexual excitement it is the secretion of the glands that enters the urethra first and ejaculates first. Next comes the glaring white secretion of the prostate gland mixed with increasing numbers of sperms, and last of all to be ejected is the thicker secretion from the seminal vesicles.

To keep the sperms alive during storage the seminal vesicles produce a kind of sugary substance similar to fruit sugar called fructose. It is this which gives semen its slightly sweet taste. Also produced is ascorbic acid (vitamin C) whence the sharp, lemony taste which many can also detect in semen. Soon after ejaculation, semen tends to semi-solidify into a firm gelatinous mass. Left for a few minutes, it re-liquefies.

**Hitting the jackpot**
The semen is deposited at the top of the vagina during intercourse, the intention of nature being fertilisation. In theory any one of his sperms is capable of fertilising each of her eggs. In practice only one sperm makes it per egg. During sexual excitement the cervix of her womb oozes a thick mucous. The semen is ejaculated onto and around this. Then, with her sexual peak which is usually immediately after male orgasm, the contractions of the uterus and the gasping and sucking of breath by her sexually excited actions cause both the mucous and semen to be drawn up some distance into the uterus. This theory has long been held and recent highly technical experiments tend to confirm it.

Sperms can live for several days after ejaculation. Their survival rate in the vagina is probably a matter of hours, but up to three days has been recorded as a survival time inside the uterus and there is no reason to regard this as the limit. The number of sperms produced is vast. It may vary up to as many as 300,000,000 per ejaculation. There are wide variations in other animals too. The dog produces three or four times as much semen as humans, the rabbit even doubles the human product, and the pig has been reported as producing a cupful or more at a time.

**Myth, magic and wet dreams**
The phenomenon of nocturnal emissions, or wet dreams, as they are more commonly called, constitutes a considerable problem to some people. Very often during sleep a man undergoes an entirely involuntary erection. This is frequently accompanied by erotic dreams. (These can be detected electrically even though they are not always remembered by the dreamer). If the excitement is enough, the wildest sexual fantasies can occur in the dreaming mind and these may culminate in a spontaneous ejaculation. At this point the dreamer usually wakes and finds himself soaked with his own cooling semen.

Apart from the inconvenience there is absolutely no harm in wet dreams. The dream is an effective overflowing and it produces marked reduction in tension. Under no conditions should it be misinterpreted. If she finds that he has had a wet dream there is no reason for her to feel guilt or dismay. Neither should he feel shame. It can happen if orgasms have been few and far between. It can also happen during a period of intense sexual excitement even if there have been repeated episodes of intercourse. It just doesn't matter. When for example, celibate priests have experienced wet dreams, both the ejaculate and in particular the vivid associated sexual dreams have tended to clash with strict religious principles. The resulting guilts can be very difficult to resolve. In past times it was commonly ordered that men undergo purifying sacrifices to dispose of the 'sin' of wet dreams! We can only repeat here that wet dreams are an entirely natural occurrence. In some men they are more frequent than in others, but either way they never constitute any danger. Anything else is utter nonsense.

There are several myths, as one might expect, about semen. In various places and times it has been held to have a magical significance. It has been used in rituals, for example, in coming-of-age ceremonies. It has been used as a fertility symbol in agricultural communities. Some primitive, tribal women regard it as a highly prestigious substance and will preserve their husbands semen if at all possible. To some creeds semen is regarded as a sort of spiritual fuel. For a man to lose it can deprive him of its value. Techniques of intercourse have been devised to bring the woman to repeated orgasm without male ejaculation for this very purpose. Even today the concept dies hard that loss of semen equates with loss of strength. Consequently many men have the idea that intercourse (or even masturbation) will tire them. Furthermore, continence is regarded as a preparation for exertion. It is true, of course, that sexual contact consumes energy,.. at a high rate even, for a short time. It is certainly true that orgasm produces a sensation of relaxation and tranquillity. Apart from that, the idea is utter rubbish. The amount of semen will be less with subsequent ejaculations and the proportion of sperms in the semen will be lower. But recovery is swift and there is no reason why the man should not orgasm several times a day without the least ill-effect if that is what he wants. With the exception of a temporarily lowered libido and perhaps a lowered intensity of excitement, there will be no other ill-effects.

**The second time around**

Many men ask, commonly as part of the general male concern over penis size, performance and so on, how long it should take them to recover. By this they mean different things and one must ask whether they mean recovery to the extent of a complete refill of the reservoirs with sperm. If so there is no exact answer. Production starts at once but could take a couple of days to complete. On the other hand sexual re-arousal seldom needs more than 20 minutes before it is possible for another bout. This period, known as the refractory period, varies from man to man and, in the same man, under differing circumstances. A survey done over a large number of men came up with the following refractory times and the percentages of men who experience them.

Men of age 20 years:

| | |
|---|---|
| Up to 5 minutes | 46% |
| 5 - 15 minutes | 38% |
| 15 - 30 minutes | 12% |
| 30 minutes and over | 4% |

Men of age 50 years

| | |
|---|---|
| Up to 5 minutes | 4% |
| 5 - 15 minutes | 11% |
| 15 - 30 minutes | 37% |
| 30 minutes and over | 48% |

I cannot confirm these figures but from my own experience I have no reason to doubt them. More recent figures have also come to hand about the actual volume of semen and number of sperms (see the work of Sobrero and Rehan, in Chicago, USA). They measured ejaculate as between 0.6 ml and a remarkable 11 ml., the average being 3.3 ml. The overall average numbers of sperms was 81 million per ml.

**Beauty and the sperm diet**

Some of the chemicals contained in semen are believed to have therapeutic value. A vague knowledge of this may have been responsible for the use of semen in the past in half-magical treatments. Chemicals known as prostaglandins are present in semen and are known to be active in a number of biochemical processes. The massaging of semen into the skin, especially of the face is highly erotic to some men and women. Many claim to have found it cosmetically useful. I have never found an explanation for this but I have encountered the story far too often from far too many reliable women to do anything other than accept it as true. Conversely, I do not believe that swallowing semen makes the breasts larger. It may be true and many people seem to think so but I personally have found no reliable evidence.

Semen can prove an inconvenient stain on clothing or upholstery, If you anticipate spilling it, try to pick the spot with a little care. If it happens anyway let it dry, then brush with a stiff brush, and sponge out with a solution of sodium bicarbonate, two teaspoons to a tumbler of luke-warm water.

**The do-it-yourself aphrodisiac**

Men might do well to remember that semen has a very slight odour that is strongly arousing to women. It has a musty, pollen-like scent and the chemicals producing that scent are similar to those in grasses and certain trees,.. notably the flowering chestnut, which is said to account for the numbers lining the streets of Paris! Hence perhaps the way that fresh mown hay is sexually exciting. Haystacks are not traditional scenes for love play simply because they are nice and springy things to lie on. More than one man I know keeps some of his own semen in a small jar in the fridge. The whole thing works and works well because of the trace quantities of pheromones that are present. These are similar to those that attract moths to mates, dogs to bitches in season and so on. The pheromones have no actual odour themselves, but a few molecules landing on the sensitive receptors of the female nose will trigger the most remarkable physiological responses,.. including an inclination for closer contact and eventually mating. A few dabs of semen behind the ears and allowed to dry before parties when followed by some cheek to cheek dancing, can have unexpected results. Perfume manufacturers beware,.. you are totally outclassed by ingenious Mother Nature!

\* \* \* \* \*

**Chapter Three:** The Psychology of the Penis

A person's final sexuality, if it is ever fair to use the word final, is a complex matter. It is not something which is wholly created and delivered with the new baby at birth ready for a lifetime of service. While some basic principles exist, the entire phenomenon of sexuality is something which is continually exposed to the varying aspects of the environment which can affect it. Development, change and response are continuous. There is seldom a time when in some small way or other progress is not being made.

Development is never ideal. Many factors are inadequately understood, or are wrongly categorised and improperly assimilated. Confused left-overs from earlier stages jostle with newly arriving thoughts and experiences. Fantasies bubble beneath the surface. The influences of art, religion and literature bias the flavours of the more primitive sexual recipe. Everyone has a slightly different sexual make-up. Everyone has a slightly different need. So, any two people coming together as potential sexual partners need to learn, understand and compromise if they are to make a success of their compatibility. Compatibility is almost never complete.

**The basic programme in the sex computer**
Sexuality has three main components. We call them genetic, intra-uterine and environmental. Between them the ever-changing 'final' stage is decided and even that goes on developing. Some characteristics of both father and mother appear in every offspring. The more obvious characteristics like colour of skin, curly hair and so on are well known to us all.

There are also some characteristics passed on from generation to generation which are not so much the original characteristics of the individual parents but those which they shared with all the other people and indeed, at a lower level, with all other animals and even all living things in general. Foremost amongst these primal instincts is the instinct for self-propagation or reproduction.

This is the so-called sex drive, a kind of innate programming designed to ensure that life goes on, that the species is reproduced and not allowed to die out with the end of the generation. To assist this all-important aim, countless other sub-programmes are built in. This is harder to show in man but apparent in animals. A female mouse, the daughter of several generations of female mice artificially inseminated with no actual contact with a male, will still react to exposure to the scent of male mouse smegma and its pheromones in a predictable way. A man shown two otherwise identical photographs of a woman in which one has had the pupils of the eyes painted in slightly larger will usually decide that the latter is the more attractive. This is an automatic response to the fact that dilated pupils signal sexual approachability. Other things which some believe to be passed on concern for example, the tendencies to homosexuality and heterosexuality. Although, as had been pointed out, celibacy is not an inherited characteristic (!), homosexuality may be, at least sometimes. This was suggested by a trial survey of twins. Where the twins were identical the majority were either both homosexual or both heterosexual. In non-identical twins the proportions were scarcely any different from the proportions to be found in the population at large.

These then are the parts of sexuality of inborn, or genetic origin. They lay down something of a sexual blueprint, a framework around which other aspects are assembled. The next big causative factor is intra-uterine influence. While a baby is growing inside its mother, for a period of some forty weeks in all, its surroundings are entirely those created by the female. The oxygen supply and food supply, indeed every requirement of the baby, comes from the mother. Its requirements are met by the baby's blood circulating into the placenta (the afterbirth). In the placenta, foods dissolved in the mother's blood pass over into the circulation of the baby. Even the warmth and safety needed are provided by the cover of the mother's protective womb and body.

At this time certain future responses are programmed into the infant. Psychologists have long been aware of the way that the typical curled-up position in which, because of the limited space available, the baby must grow, becomes, in later life, a position of comfort and rest often chosen for relaxation and sleep as well as for instinctive actions of protection. Another influence of great importance is the heart rate and breathing rate of the mother. Certain emotions in the mother change the very nearby pulsating rhythms of her heart. At the same time chemicals like adrenalin may be released into her own circulation, thus changing it slightly. Some of these changes are witnessed by the baby too. Even more significant are the hormones of the mother. Hormones, the product of a group of small but very important endocrine glands, are chemicals released into the bloodstream. The amounts produced are out of all proportion to their enormous effects. Minute quantities can cause dramatic responses.

One such group of chemicals are the so-called sex hormones. During the whole intra-uterine period when there is no influence from the father's hormones, the baby is subjected to a special little world provided exclusively by the mother. As yet we do not know the details of what effects this has, but it is not hard to appreciate that it must be capable of the most profound influences. Modern experiments are probing this largely unexplored field. What we all know is that women exist in infinite variety. The extremes of exceedingly timid, retiring, 'traditionally female' women and the opposites of dominant, short-haired masculine women who shave twice a week exist in all communities. At least in part these differences are hormone influenced. The differing effects of the 'hormone bath' of the intra-uterine life with its varying degrees of maleness and femaleness are not so far understood. They unquestionably exist.

**First impressions last forever**

As soon as the baby is born a whole new set of influences start to affect it. Compressed by the walls of the very organ that has been its home, the infant is squeezed during the course of a few hours down a narrow and constricting tube. The pressures put on it are enough to move the fragile, gristly bones of its skull until they overlap. Then finally, within seconds, the entire new human is ejected quite violently into the outside world. Its body feels cold and is simultaneously subjected to intense light, neither of these having been experienced before. The shock helps galvanise the chest and lungs into life. For the first time air is sucked into the lungs. The tiny heart changes its action as the umbilical cord, the all-important life-line to the mother is severed. The whole circulation makes a monumental change for the one and only time in its life. All this happening within such a short space of time has an understandably shocking effect. More is to come.

On a mental and emotional level the Jesuit priests, a militant order of the Catholic religion, had long-since recognised the importance of early events on the eventual individual. Ideas and lessons rubbed in during the first six or eight years of life seem virtually indelible. They get into the memory without any adequate censorship being imposed by the young recipient. Discipline ensures adherence. Rewards or punishments reinforce the acceptance of the ideas. Much of the grown man exists at least as a pattern by the age of seven.

It is during these years too that the sexuality is powerfully influenced, often irrevocably. Such factors as the domination level of parents, their attitudes to sex, the school control of sexual differences and so on all leave their imprint on the expanding mind. Some workers claim to have detected a statistical association between babies who were breast-fed and adults who are 'bosom' men or breast influenced, that is, who are more than ordinarily excited on by breasts as sex objects. Some even claim to recognise the placing of the baby on rubber waterproof bedding as associated with a tendency towards rubber fetishism in later years. All that is known for sure is that these very early years go far in presenting the eventual sexuality of the individual. It is my own feeling that little that happens after the first ten years causes any major change. Minor variations, learning and experimenting may well occur, but in all likelihood no radical rearrangements of sexuality happen after the first decade. If someone allegedly becomes homosexual at the age of forty, I believe they were homosexual at the age of ten at the latest and were in the interim, acting out a heterosexual phase. (The question of bi-sexuality in relation to this is discussed elsewhere).

**The sexual phase**
Whatever are the individual causes and effects, in broad outline the developing sexuality of the infant is in phases which, although overlapping at either end, are nonetheless distinguishable. A new-born male child will commonly undergo an erection during its first few minutes of life. In some cultures this is regarded as forecasting a strong virile man to come. Whatever anyone says to the contrary there is little doubt that this practice does take place in many places. Even in UK I have met midwives who believe such an erection should be encouraged with a little gentle masturbation. Elsewhere it is the task of another woman, usually the babe's mother, to suck the infant penis erect if it does not spontaneously become stiff.

I have encountered this in UK too and have always seen it as a harmless part of the mother-and-child bonding process. It is indeed very strongly emotional for some women though I often suspect this is more a feature of mother-love than of any sexual content. Of course, in earlier, and perhaps better times, the question of abuse was less likely to be the interpretation of such actions than would be the case today. I think there are possible pitfalls though I do not think I could go as far as to regard such maternally affectionate actions as being in any way deemed to be encouraging any form of anti-social behaviour. Indeed, I am of the opinion that such actions do not in any way constitute so-called 'sexual abuse.' I suspect that if the practice is ever curtailed on the grounds of being a form of abuse, then losses will outweigh gains. It is certain that even without any outside help, during washing and powdering and so on plenty of babies, male and female, commonly become obviously sexually excited and will make movements which in the adult are clearly discernible as associated with copulation and orgasm.

**Oral, anal and asexual**
In general, the first stage of sexuality, lasting up to about eighteen months, is the oral phase. Pleasures tend to result from such things as sucking and gaining nourishment. As it grows the baby will put things in its mouth partly to touch and get to know them and

partly because there is pleasure in mouth stimulation. Following on is the phase to which much pleasure has been allocated, the anal phase. At this time, from say one year to three years, the anus and rectum seem to dominate the sexual scene. Erection may accompany defecation. The profound effects of 'potty training' to which society attaches such importance are felt at this stage.

Next comes the phallic stage lasting until perhaps six years. There is frequent and prolonged masturbation. Although the child is not aware of the significance of sexuality, its impulses are so strong that it will fondle its genitalia in public or, for example, rub itself against another person, commonly the mother. While these actions are innocent from the child's viewpoint, they are embarrassing to the conditioned (and often confused) minds of the adults. Admonishment may result, which in its turn, confuses the infant too. The vicious circle starts its next round.

Between about five years and twelve years there is a so-called latent phase sexually. Little of a sexual nature seems to interest or concern the child. Nothing much in the way of experiment takes place until, with the first onset of earliest puberty, there is a re-birth of interest. The opposite sex becomes a subject of mixed fear and fascination. Masturbation in earnest begins. The final, genital phase of developing sexuality has arrived.

**Discovering life's most fascinating toy**
To define gender accurately in a way that will satisfy everyone is not easy. A good working definition is that it is the sum of the peculiarities of structure and function that distinguish a male from a female. Whatever are the origins and biological facts one of the most obvious of those 'peculiarities' is that he has a penis, and she doesn't. Seeing a young sister who has no penis has affected many a little boy with an anxious fear that he might lose his. At around five or six perhaps, when the lad is at the height of his Oedipus confusion, seeing his father's comparatively large and threatening penis can start the development of a feeling of jealousy and competition with father and indeed brothers and men in general. There is also a security phenomenon perhaps related originally to the idea that plenty (of food, clothing, shelter, etc.) equates with safety. Big is beautiful and biggest is best is only another sign of the acquisition of property inclination of mankind in general. Furthermore the penis is nice. It swells, does interesting things, is a secret, feels good, impresses girls (and boys) and so on. Small wonder that in the developing mind of the child, the penis, for a whole series of reasons, starts to become very important.

Little if anything ever happens to reduce this significance. The penis continues as a source of awe, excitement, comfort and, as it grows, pride. Long before the far higher significance of style and technique become apparent it is size that matters. The worst thing that could happen would be to have no penis at all (hence castration fears). The next worse thing is to have a poor, miserable, pathetic, little winkle. The best thing is to have a monstrous-looking creature capable of swift arousal to a long, thick, vibrant shaft supporting a glistening red head as tight and as big as a baby's fist with a crab apple in it! The scene is set and the play begins, which, throughout a man's life, will have deep significance. However big, the man wishes his penis bigger, however long, longer would be better, however sturdy, wider would be an improvement. To him it follows from this reasoning that in this way he can be at least as good and maybe even better than his father and other men. It follows too, he feels, that women will be impressed, dominated, thrilled and kept faithful by the huge pleasure-giver/punisher that lurks beneath the trouser zip! Such is the actual if distorted and disproportionate view hidden in the depths of the male psyche.

**Penis size and sexual power**

The arguments of women who say that it is performance rather than size that matters most are irrelevant to men. We are not talking about a totally logical situation. Nothing will ever convince the average man that big is not best. It is true to say, in fact, that, even for those women who so fervently declare the unimportance of penis size, much of their comment arises from lack of experience. Few women have ever been penetrated by a really tiny or a really huge penis. Many have experience of only half a dozen penises anyway. It may be true that there is scant difference between a seven inch penis and a seven and a half inch penis, or even between a five inch one and a seven inch one. However, intercourse with a three inch long, index-finger midget or a twelve inch organ of near three inch diameter, is an experience given to few ladies. Those who have such experience tell a different story. As a rule neither extreme meets with much appreciation.

Size does matter and within limits it quite certainly does matter immensely to women too. The comment of the experienced woman is usually that although other things like skill and care for their feelings matter a great deal, when all other things are equal, the larger penis is the more appreciated. And there, in a nutshell, is the significant factor of all the prolonged discussions on the relevance of penis size. The majority of women will answer the same thing,.. better a good, big one than a good little one. That is what is known for certain and that is all that needs to be known. Men and women alike, perhaps for different reasons, prefer a big penis to a small one.

Most of all though, penis size matters to a man. It is one of his great pride centres. Much of his ego is in, or is at least supported by, his penis. As long as men think, wish and hope that the size of the penis really counts, then it does. That is the be-all and end-all of the argument. Their minds are made up. It is useless confusing them with facts. The whole thing speaks for itself. Men have decided, believed and been conditioned into a way of thinking that accepts penis size as of supreme relevance. So there all fruitful discussion and argument might as well end. If men are convinced that it counts,.. it does.

**The lunatic fringe**

Adult sexual behaviour is governed by four separate but overlapping groups of influences. These are neurological (the essential nerve control of sexual function, libido, etc.) endocrinological (the working of the sex hormone and other chemical-producing glands), psychological, and sociological (the effect of currently accepted ideals, principles, taboos etc.). It is in the latter areas that the question of penis-size arises. It is here too that the misguided ideas and confusions of earlier generations have their lingering effect.

About a hundred years ago, on the tenth of August, 1898 in San Francisco, USA, was issued Patent No.587994. It was for a male chastity belt. Men could wear these or lock their sons into one. The padded steel and leather belt anchored firmly about the waist and thighs. The penis passed through a ring or short cylinder to reach the outside world. The rings and cylinders were specially equipped. Even the slightest erection meant that a series of pins prodded deeply into the shaft of the penis. The aim of the device was to 'stop nocturnal emission, control waking thoughts, and prevent self-abuse.' Great thinking, you might comment. How quaint such ideas would be if they were not so barbaric. How wrong and confused people were,.. back in those days.

But it is as well to be vigilant. Such mentalities abound amongst us,.. in the red-neck, fundamentalist and politically extreme right-wings, for example. Be warned,.. bizarre mental processes are not all that far below the surface of a lot of the minds you will pass on the way to the office this very day.

\* \* \* \* \*

## Chapter Four: Penis Technique

In any sexual encounter, there are three guiding principles that separate the skilled and caring participant from the unskilled, clumsy ignoramus. They apply equally to men and women.

1. Aim to please your partner as well as yourself. This involves vast amounts of study, practice, perseverance and open-mindedness. It is one of the finest of all human ideals to be co-operative and helpful at a sexual level. If you haven't already learned, whatever your age, it's never too late to start if you have enough motivation. And it's always worth it. It may prove especially difficult for older people who have become rather set and inflexible in their ways and ideas. This should be recognised as a distinct threat to a continued relationship. There is much that can and should be done about the situation. Several excellent books on the subject exist, in particular *'Age and Sex'* by Dr.Richard Silurian (See Sources List).

2. Do what you like and don't do what you don't like (except in the interest of No.1)

3. Nothing is wrong between lovers short of actual injury, so long as both want it. There can be a variety of reasons, not all of them sexual, why they might want whatever they want. It must be mentioned that in some places and at some times some sexual practices have been and are still illegal. For example all male homosexual anal intercourse used to be illegal in England and in some American states. Nowadays, anal intercourse between adult males in private has been made legal in England,.. however precisely the same act between loving husband and wife continued to be forbidden for years after it became so. It remains forbidden in many other places. It is hard to locate the logic herein. When such archaic and illogical laws exist whereby heterosexual anal intercourse could still constitute grounds for divorce,.. then it is the laws that need changing, not the practice.

It should not be inferred from these three basic rules that there is not a place for the sudden, swift and selfish sexual episode. Quickies, as they are often called, can be a lot of fun for the giver and the receiver. Some people find it a very powerful initial turn-on to have a short sex bout when they have to be hasty, or careful not to be found out, or both. But here we are concerned with the detailed and dedicated approach to sexual acts and in particular to the function of the penis therein.

**Erotic acrobats**

The variations of penis function depend to some extent on the different positions of intercourse. Here at once we are into a matter that has produced some of the greatest discussion, speculation and wasted time in history. I'm not sure what the record is but at least one classification has in excess of six hundred positions. Many of them are only minutely different from others, mere angles of the eyes sufficing to produce the difference.

In the same way, perhaps, as one can be a connoisseur of fine wines, it must be conceded that vast experience can probably enable a man to be aware of such subtleties. I calculate however that it would probably require at least three sexual encounters per day from the age of fifteen to around fifty-five to acquire such qualifications. Only the most stalwart could survive the ordeal and remain coherent. Furthermore, so many of the positions appear to have been designed for creatures other than human,.. those having six joints in each leg might be more suitable. For those of us restricted to the customary hip, knee and ankle, to remain poised, while in a state of sexual excitement in some of the more elaborate figures and for anything above a few seconds would not only require contortionism but would perhaps have a negative effect on the entire enjoyment of sex as well as upon the sustained physical health and ability to continue it; the sound of arches falling and hernias slipping could probably be heard for three blocks.

**The basic choices**

All this is said to poke fun at the purists who concern themselves with such nonsense. For, in principle, there are only two main directions from which the penis can enter the vagina: from the front, and from the rear. Each of these directions can be sub-divided into two types: straight and not-straight. That's all there is to it apart from the picturesque but unhelpful, poetic ways in which the Orientals of history named the positions.

When the penis contacts the vagina, there are really only two things it can do apart from remaining motionless. It can go inside and rub or it can stay outside and rub. This latter is sometimes known by the Americanism of 'high-riding.' Consider that the woman is lying on her back, her legs parted enough to allow her partner to lie between them. Instead of inserting the glans into the vagina, he lays its undersurface in the groove formed by the front portion of the vulval cleft, where the lips come together and, making movements of his pelvis, rubs it backwards and forwards in the crease. The most sensitive part of the penis (the undersurface of the glans) is now against the most sensitive part of the female genitalia, the clitoris. Lubricated, if necessary, the friction is now varied in pressure, speed, the length of the rubbing, and to an extent in direction. The glans will quickly rub its way down between the lips, separating them and leaving the clitoris exposed to the action. When aroused this erects and bulges out. Though it is very small, and difficult to think of in this way, its own 'undersurface' which is also the most sensitive, is the part most affected. This high-riding is, for some people, an extremely erotic sensation. Some women prefer it to actual penetration. By having her head and shoulders up on pillows and by him using his arms to lever himself clear of the woman, they can both also watch the glans as it slithers, first towards their eyes, then away again. Both can detect the subtle movements of greatest sensation and anticipate them both. Both too can watch ejaculation over the woman's mons and abdomen. As the shaft of the penis is scarcely if at all compressed, the semen may well squirt powerfully and a long way up. Many couples find this to be a highly significant and symbolic act.

At this point it is as well to put in a word about lubrication. There is a widely held and largely inaccurate idea amongst men that women produce lubrication in vast quantities. Some think they actually 'come' a liquid something like semen at orgasm. They don't. Very few produce much in the way of 'juices.' Indeed, most of the 'juices' seen afterwards are simply leaking semen. So unless you are one of those rare girls who produce unusual amounts you may be glad of some extra help. A man too should understand that women vary in this characteristic. Even the same woman may vary in the amount she produces at different stages of her life and even at different times of the month. This means that some extra lubrication can be an essential. Invariably, saliva is the most handy. A penis just out of the partner's mouth is fine, or some extra saliva may be transferred by hand. But one has to be a little careful where that hand has been, in the interests of hygiene. Some people use Vaseline but it is greasy and hard to wash off afterwards. KY Jelly is better but, being water-based, it tends to dry and become tacky too soon and you may need to add more during the proceedings. Nivea Cream or any good hand or body lotion is best of all.

NOTE: Some condoms are made of materials that are swiftly damaged by oily lubricants. If you are using that type avoid oils. There are plenty of condoms available which are pre-lubricated with oil and do not so deteriorate.

**Invention is the mother of pleasure**

The vulva is not the only place for using the penis. Some will enjoy the penis rubbing up between the buttocks. This is best done by placing her on her knees with her thighs far enough apart for him to kneel between them. He kneels very close to her, places his penis almost upright between her cheeks and rubs. She, looking back between her legs sees the testicles dangling and moving and can enjoy the sensation of them against her. He sees the action very clearly, and both have the erotic sensation that can arise from the penis stroking over the back part of the vaginal lips, the perineum and its hair, and, in particular, over the sensitive area of the anal orifice.

Another way is to place the penis in the fold of the groin. This can be one from on top or from the side. She, in particular, may enjoy lying flat, face up or down, with the penis tightly trapped between her closed thighs and/or vulval lips. Suitably positioned, she can also play with its glans as it emerges on each thrust. The erotic effects of high-riding, on women more especially, have to be indulged in to be appreciated. They can be colossal. There is also an advantage accruing from the fact that, proceeding to orgasm, the semen is not squirted into the vagina. As one wit put it, doing this out of doors, can result in 'casting your seed on stony ground.' The point is that the further away from the vulva it goes the less the chance of pregnancy. Pregnancy is possible without actually putting the semen in the vagina, but, as perhaps the same wit might have put it, it's a pretty long shot. Don't rely on it as a contraceptive technique.

Man is the only higher animal to make love face to face. Man's anatomy makes a wider choice of sexual positions available to him. He tends to enjoy great variation. He doesn't adopt the mere strict biological aspects of sex but adapts and extends them for additional pleasures. Not all people everywhere and always have used the same position as their most customary position. If the story is true, it was only after watching male white missionaries bringing other than purely ecclesiastical benefits to local, native girls that some African tribes and South Sea Islanders named the 'normal' white European [man on top] position as the 'Missionary' way. What amused them about the method was not so much the fact that it was a face-to-face variety of intercourse, but that it was the woman lying on her back with the man on top doing the work. In their way, the man relaxed on his back while the woman squatted over him and made the necessary efforts. Other allegedly more primitive peoples prefer rear entry in common with other mammals. All positions have certain advantages.

**A connoisseur's guide to intercourse**

Face to face intercourse with the woman supine, that is, on her back, is the first choice of a large percentage of women. The reasons given are many. Two explanations exist. The first is conditioning. It is what they are used to. It is comfortable. It feels right, natural and safe. Equally important is that in this position the pressure on the clitoris is at its greatest. The man's hard ridge of bone across the abdomen above the root of the penis (called the pubic bone) presses against the area of the clitoris. It crushes against it the crisp male pubic hair, and indeed that of the female. In and out movements alternately pull and relax the labia and with them the foreskin of the clitoris. It is this pressure, rubbing and pulling that produces the sensation, more so, usually, than the movement of the penis within the vagina.

One other factor is significant. The penis, especially of the younger man, stands not only out but up. In most women it is the front (anterior) wall of the vagina that is the most sensitive. When she is supine, especially with her thighs down and a pillow under her hips, the probing penis presses hardest and most pleasurably against this wall. During intercourse it is a good idea to reach down, pull the labia apart in front to expose the clitoris more completely, then put the weight fully down upon it thus keeping the labia from coming together again. As she approaches her orgasm he can lift his feet and lower legs or even, with practice, his knees and thighs too. By gripping hard around her shoulders or on a convenient bed edge, he can ride her such that the lowest part of him touching anything is his pubic bone. The great pressure can be much appreciated. But try it gently until you're sure of your partner's feelings. Somebody said that you can define a gentleman as someone who, during intercourse, always takes the weight on his elbows. By no means all women agree. Many enjoy the man's weight. It's all a matter of preference.

Face to face positions have other advantages. There is someone to talk to if that's what you like. There are breasts to look at and play with, though this is not always easy when lying. Breasts are attractive to all men, for some exclusively so. These men tend to prefer face to face positions. Visibility however is limited and if seeing things is important then other alternatives are more successful. By kneeling up and spreading her legs wide he can get a better view down onto his penetrating penis. The aroma of the genitalia will drift up to his nostrils and his extended hands can grasp and fondle the breasts. Variations in the angle of penetration can be achieved by the size and position of pillows under her. Under her buttocks they tilt her pelvis up, under the small of her back down. He should never forget, whichever way he has penetrated, that he can make the penis touch different spots in the vagina by changing his hip and thrusting angle. Or he can grasp the penis root in his hand and move it accordingly. Also, if kneeling up, he can manipulate the clitoris rather than merely rub it with his pubis. Lifting her thighs at varying degrees including until her knees are beside her ears (be gentle until you know how far they'll go) also changes the degree of pressure against different parts of the vaginal orifice.

Having her on top, the so-called 'woman-superior' positions for instance, while still face to face, has the same and additional benefits. For example, if he is very heavy, or if for any reason, such as after surgery or illness, deep penetration is unwelcome. Kneeling or squatting astride him, she has choice of timing and ferocity and also controls the depth to which she is penetrated. She can rub her own clitoris either with a finger or against her partner. Though a large proportion of women prefer intercourse on their backs, there is no doubt that the second largest group prefer it this way. It has an appeal for him too in that he can pass his hands around her buttocks and freely feel the movements of his penis. And he can increase her stimulation by stroking her labia and her anus.

As mentioned above the alternative to straight face to face intercourse is non-straight. This is also known as *'flanquette.'* The only important difference is that instead of his legs being between hers, they are astride one or other of them. Correspondingly hers must be astride one of his. There is only one apparent benefit from this position apart from being a mere change. Different areas of skin, in particular the inner surfaces of the thighs, come into contact with the partner's skin. You have only to try it to find it pleasantly novel. Similarly, the angle of entry into the vagina is different.

The other main group of intercourse positions is from the rear, positions also called *'croupade.'* The number of women preferring rear entry is smaller than those preferring front entry, though the percentage increases during the fourth and even more so in the fifth and sixth decades. Reasons given vary but common amongst them is that it makes her feel less personal. Somehow she feels more 'used' than treated as an individual. Some women mistakenly imagine that as it's only her bottom he can see it could be anyone's. This is not true. There is told in medical circles the story of the gynaecologist who entered the operating theatre when the first of his patients was already anaesthetised and waiting for him. Her face was covered by the anaesthetic mask but her genitalia were washed and exposed ready for his attention. He glanced at them and said, "Ah, it's Mrs. Smith first I see." This should convince any lady that she is as distinctive there as she in on her face, and every bit as attractive. It's just that she doesn't see that area often herself. Rear entry can be effected by the penis with her standing, touching her toes, kneeling, lying or having her legs well astride. He should bear in mind certain essentials in each instance. Standing, she will need steadying in order not to fall; in case things get carried away it's as well to have something soft for her to fall on anyway. Touching her toes she is even more likely to overbalance. Kneeling, is most women's preferred choice.

Rear entry with her kneeling is high on the male list of favourites too. For the large proportion of men who are 'bottoms' men, it presents a superb view of the buttocks, the gap between, and the anus. The view of the active penis is at its best. The depth of penetration is the greatest. In fact, he should be careful as he can easily be far enough in to press against a nearby ovary. An ovary is as tender to pressure as a testicle. His hands are free to spread her or stroke her. He can reach around in front to play with her breasts. As her degree of sensation is likely to be reduced by the lack of clitoral involvement he should always give this some attention. It is also valuable if he withdraws the penis and runs it up and down her crease and against her clitoris from time to time. If she looks back at this stage she can also watch ejaculation if it is not to be internal.

For some girls the somewhat limited physical pleasure can be improved by a psychological one. If he grasps her wrists and holds them behind her she has the feeling of being pinioned and 'taken.'

Or it is possible for her to kneel astride him as he lies on his back, her face towards his feet. The position of the penis in this position is to push hard up onto the back or posterior wall of the vagina. Its movement causes the anus to be stretched and relaxed at each push. If he likes that, the view is second to none and a penetrating finger can further improve matters. Rear entry is also ideal for 'lazy' intercourse. For this, both are lying on their sides. It is perfect for when he wants it and she wants to sleep, or already is asleep perhaps just distantly feeling his affectionate movements within her.

The only alternative to straight rear entry is non-straight. This is called *'cuissade.'* As with frontal non-straight entry, the only difference is being astride the partner's thighs instead of being between or astride them both. Again it is the angle of the penis in the vagina and the different skin surfaces touching that provide the thrill.

A question often asked at sex-counselling clinics concerns the use of contraceptives by the male. There is only one effective male contraceptive, and even that is not perfect. It is best known as the condom,.. or sheath, protective cover, French letter or, more graphically the rubber overcoat. Most are well made of quality latex materials and thoroughly tested. Their inefficiency comes mostly from misuse and bad handling. They do reduce contact and sensation but some users enjoy the 'kinky' feel of rubber. They also vastly reduce the spread of venereal disease and AIDS.

When, then, should a condom be put on? There is only one answer not dictated by personal preference and that is before you lose control and can't hold back. If you're not sure then sooner is better than later. There are only two ways of putting it on. One is to fumble furtively and secretly. The only place for this is during a questionable seduction routine. The other way is openly, even blatantly and with a flourish. He should kneel up and unroll it down the penis shaft while letting the penis jut towards her almost as if in threat. If she is ready this will turn her up, not down. If she's not ready he probably shouldn't be doing it anyway. It is usually much appreciated if she puts it on for him. But a few words of warning. Although it goes easier onto a wet penis it is far better put on a dry one. It doesn't slip off so easily. And put it on straight. Askew, the penis can tear it. After ejaculation don't leave the sheathed penis in the vagina to go soft. You may lose the sheath. By the way, it's nothing to be frightened of if you do lose it. Two searching fingers can usually grasp it. If he or she can't, a doctor can next day. It can't go anywhere else apart from falling out, though I have heard of this happening in somewhat embarrassing circumstances,.. the girl in question having been too ashamed to visit a certain supermarket ever since.

No discussion of the penis in relation to the vagina is complete without a discussion of performance. A few questions and answers may help. How far should he go in? The answer is as far as he wants to without hurting her; or, put another way, as far as she can allow and she wants him to. A big penis will enter a small woman as long as it is done gently. Sharply stabbing in a big dry penis and thrusting it home to the hilt is stupid and painful and is not likely to be met with any gratitude or amorous response. But lubricated and gently penetrating, it can go a little further each time and the wonderful muscles of the vagina will relax and stretch. Remember a baby's head comes out through the vagina with remarkably little difficulty and however big the penis is, it won't be that big.

How long should intercourse continue? Again it's choice that matters. The more you do it, the more chance of making her sore and him too. She may also get a troublesome irritation of the bladder next day. Anything up to an hour, if he can manage it, shouldn't hurt anyone. There is no harm in approaching orgasm, holding it back to let it settle, then having another crescendo or so. There is no harm in not having an orgasm at all. It might be a bit disappointing but no-one suffers. Prolonging intercourse is just a matter of co-operative and extensive training for both partners. Details of this training are given later in The Broken Penis section. Suffice it to say at this stage that if he or she comes too soon too often, they are badly in need of more time, effort and practice as enjoyable sexual sessions are being unnecessarily curtailed to the benefit of no-one.

Finally how many times? Again the answer is as many as you like. Some monks and nuns allegedly almost never orgasm. Some men and women do it several times a day. It's only in the mind that sex 'tires you out.' If you believe intercourse in the morning will tire you, it will seem to do so. Left alone you should recharge pretty quickly though it may reduce your interest for later in the day. (Some people say you should not have intercourse in the morning because you never know who you might meet later on!) However, a good woman can usually use her feminine charms effectively to bring a man on again if she needs him. Also, if she is the one who hasn't yet recharged, she can at least make herself available for him if he needs her.

* * *

**Chapter Five:** The Penis Elsewhere

Whether you think that variety is the spice of life or that spice is the life of variety, most people would agree that variety is vitally important to interest and enjoyment. Man goes to endless lengths to produce variety. Even the most routine-loving of people have some areas in which they enjoy a change. The majority of us like plenty of change. All of man's natural functions have been subjected to the search for greater variety. Eating and drinking are supreme examples.

Our actual requirements for nourishment are astonishingly simple. Apart from traces of a few chemicals, we need only water to drink. Cooking is nothing but the blending of colours, flavours and textures and the application of heat. Yet each combination and its aromas that exist in the Cordon Bleu world finds an appreciative palate. Protection from the elements is, in many climates, an essential, but the spectrum of fashions has far exceeded even the wildest requirements of that function. Even breathing has been pressed into service as a pleasure source by the habit of smoking and the use of fragrant perfumes and incenses. It would be odd for a person not to acquire a large and changing variety of interests and preferences during a lifetime. Though some may remain largely static, others are sure to alter.

It is against this background that sexual variety should also be seen. Sex, which is one of man's most intrinsic natural functions, has at least the same ability for variety built into it as does eating. It would thus be equally unnatural and illogical for anyone to develop a rigidly fixed attitude about it. Yet it does happen. Often as a result of the existence of false but restrictive taboos, sex, in some places and some times, gets singled out for a disproportionately different treatment. Such a period has just come to its end with the passing of the sexually hypocritical Victorian/Edwardian phase of Western society. That passing has left a lot of outmoded, even vicious ideas high and dry. A radical re-thinking has become necessary. It takes time.

One of the things about sex that has been sadly in need of such re-thinking for a long while is the whole question of sexual variations, deviations and perversions. Reading the work of earlier writers, it seems to me that there was frequently a tendency to describe any particular sexual practice not enjoyed by the writer as being a perversion,.. while one's own particular perversions are regarded as mere deviations! It is a very difficult problem because the kind of sex one doesn't enjoy, as often as not doesn't just leave one cold, it frankly repels. This is in part a habit, and a bad habit.

**One man's meat is another man's perversion**
The first requirement of understanding is to realise that before there can be a perversion of, or a deviation from, the normal there has to be a normal. And there isn't. The nearest one can get to normal would be a 'here and now' normal. In today's world the here and now changes with such rapidity as to make such generalisations dubious and unhelpful. If you must have a definition of perversion try this one. Sexual perversion is the repeated substitution for a sexual practice of an ultimately non-sexual behaviour process. Nothing short of that can be described as perverse, only as differing degrees of variation. There is nothing more odd about a man who enjoys having his penis rubbed with cold cream than there is about a woman who has a great fondness for devouring the boiled entrails of a pig. There is nothing more queer about a woman who likes to be tied to the bed and masturbated than there is about a man who enjoys spending his Saturday

evenings throwing little pointed bits of metal at a circular piece of cork on a bar-room wall.

Sexual variation and preferences develop through life. Basic trends are often detectable and these seldom change radically. Rather, there is a tendency to try new things and discard them, retain them for occasional use, or make them a part of the favoured routine. A person's sexual preferences are highly individual. They are a basic feature of the person,.. and being such they are ignored only with the greatest potential hazard.

It is impossible to love someone totally without regarding their sex as loveable too. Where two individuals love and live together there are thousands of places where their differences can provide sources of friction. Part of the whole point is in overcoming, compromising and compensating for the frictions. Nowhere is this more important than with sexual variations. Some things a couple will enjoy in common and do often. Other things they will do just for the enjoyment of helping each other. A woman will do extra washing to save on the laundry and buy her man a new CD for his car. He will do unwelcome overtime to buy her new curtains. He will give her the anal intercourse she craves though it affords him no particular excitement. She will suck him off although it gives her only limited sexual pleasure. Life is, or should be, like that; the wise and thoughtful will seek out the preferences and provide them unasked, for the sheer pleasure of it. Try and go along if you can, willingly and helpfully, never, never, by coercion and with dragging feet. Say no if you must but realise what you are doing. An atmosphere of sexual wantonness is a great gift,.. to give is to receive.

**Armpit**
Putting the penis into an armpit is a strong turn-on for some men. Shaven smooth, prickly short stubble or bushy hair all have their adherents. Perhaps the scent helps too. There are two ways. One way the penis lies in the fold of the armpit from front to back or vice versa. The other way is to kneel astride the chest and push the knob up into the armpit. She then folds her upper arm to trap it against her ribs or breast. This position provides the knob with a surface to press against with the thrusts.

**Breasts**
An even greater favourite is to fuck the breasts. If he is kneeling astride her, both can get a lot of sensation from rubbing the under surface of the penis over an erect nipple. If she is uppermost she can dangle her nipples against him. Alternatively, stroking his penis with her cascading hair, her tongue and her nipples, can lead on to trapping the penis between her breasts and massaging it up and down. She may be able to reach it with a tongue-tip at the upper extremity of its movement. One thing she must be careful about as with any long-stroke working of the penis,.. don't pull the foreskin too far back, especially the underneath part. It hurts.

**Voyeurism**
Lots of people like to make love in the dark. To lie in a warm bed covered with blankets in a cocoon of darkness is said by the psychologists to create a safe, womb-like environment which nearly everyone finds comforting. It may also help to overcome shyness. But one of nature's powerful weapons of attraction is vision. That's why peacocks have tails and men have beards. To some, not seeing is almost as bad as not doing.

There are two varieties of voyeurism. The true voyeur (or voyeuse) gets the kicks from watching others make love. There is always a fascinated group by the baboon cage in the zoo if they are at it! Whether or not you like watching others, it is certainly a first class way to learn. If one picture is worth a thousand words, one 'dirty' picture is worth at least a hundred fumbles. Even from a blue movie you can learn a lot, especially some of the more imaginative, top-class, so-called hard core material. Best of all is to watch a really capable and experienced couple make love. It's a pity such opportunities so seldom arise. Of course the thought is still shocking to some but one of the few reasons for getting into a group sex scene is to get involved with older, more experienced types and to listen, watch and learn,.. even if you don't actually take part for reasons of personal preference or hygiene.

More commonly, voyeurism describes the desire to watch oneself or one's partner. This is quite a different matter. It is an adjunct to one's sex life, perhaps a favoured part of it; but it is not a substitute for it. Happily there is something of the voyeur in everyone. Unless there is a serious hitch, even the most demure of girls is likely to find some things appealing to look at. So what can he do? It has to be admitted that Nature and Fashion have not been exactly liberal in distributing ways in which the undressed man (as opposed to the fully dressed one) can appear sexy. His object must therefore be to fascinate.

It is possible for a man to undress sexily, but only just. (Perhaps the best, all-too-brief portrayal of disastrous disrobing is in the movie '*A Fish Called Wanda*'). The very first rule of all, never to be broken, is shoes and socks off first. Nothing is more macabre than a man sitting on the edge of the bed and fumbling to get his shoes undone when his trousers are already down around his ankles. No man with any heart would make love with his socks on,.. it's like sleeping in your vest or picking your nose with gloves on. There are only two things a man can take off that are the least bit sexy. If he wears a tie he can undo it slowly and unbutton his shirt. The other thing is his belt. Particularly if it is a large, heavy belt, undoing it very deliberately is not without its appeal. At this stage he will often have at least a half-erected penis bulging his trousers. Tilting the pelvis forward as he unzips will draw her attention to the bulge. At the last moment he should slip the trousers and pants low enough at the front to let the penis protrude. It will hold her interest long enough for him to complete the ungainly action of dropping the trousers. These should now be stepped out of or kicked aside, never picked up and neatly folded. (When he is dressing afterwards, assuming he is ever coming back to the same lady, he should never be careless. Don't leave her with the visual, romantic memory of you in your shirt-tail and socks groping for a shoe under the bed.

The uncircumcised man might next pull back the foreskin and press down at the root of the penis against the pubic bone. This sharpens the angle at which it juts out and also retains blood so that it assumes an even larger proportion and more aggressive appearance. He might now put her hand on it or merely offer it to her. He might show it to her right up close where the scent of it, with those naturally erotically evocative pheromones, can reach her. There comes a point where no book on sex can help and you are on your own. Remember a couple of useful tips. Girls like to dress up and be appreciated. So, if she puts on her sexy gear for you, make a point of appreciating. Watch throughout as carefully as you can. Apart from the sexual pleasures of voyeurism, observation will reveal a dozen little clues to her likes and dislikes. She may be too shy to tell you and visual reactions may be your only guide.

This latter is just as useful advice for her. When it comes to voyeurism though, this is one game in which she dictates the bulk of the play. All men like to see but for those in whom seeing is a highly developed preference it places immense strength at her disposal. A man will return again and again to a woman whose visual efforts please him even when she is ageing or has lost much of her physical charm. To start with it can be difficult for a woman unused to 'indecency' to expose herself openly. But it is more natural to show than to hide. The showing instinct is built-in, the hiding habit is tacked on by conditioning. Given a fair chance instinct will always triumph.

So learn what he likes to see you in. Whether it's just your jewellery, or a mini-skirt, or your black boots makes no difference. He's chosen you and you've chosen him so why not choose the gear that matches? Learn to display yourself. Don't hesitate to bend over, or lie on the bed in the position he likes. If he likes it lift up your legs and open them, open your lips brazenly, and let him look at the places that draw him. It doesn't hurt a bit. You must assess the man carefully. Some, far from liking it, will feel threatened by too 'whorish' an exposure. Again at some point you're on your own. But he knows you dress up to go out, so why shouldn't you dress up to stay in with him? After all, for whom do you dress up? If for him, it's illogical not to seize every chance to wear the things he likes.

**On reflection**

Voyeurism can be further developed by the use of mirrors. One or two in the bedroom will give either or both the chance to watch if they want. And again it doesn't hurt. Some couples get a turn-on from reading sexy books or looking at sexy pictures. This also offers a chance to learn, partly from the pictures and partly from seeing what the other likes. "Show me what you like, darling, so I can do it for you" is an under-used, underestimated key to sexual bliss. You might try writing each other detailed sexy letters. One couple I know exchange letters before he goes away on his business trips. Then the night before he comes home they talk on the phone if possible and tell each other exactly what they're going to do. They are in their late fifties and no wonder they're so fit and happy,.. and still so head-over-heels in love! An orgasm a day keeps the doctor away,.. and it's much more fun than apples!

**Oral sex**

This is a subject that seems to be causing a great deal of unnecessary confusion. I have even been asked by a learned judge in a court if it was something people really did. The answer is, yes they do. Who? Almost anyone who can, or who has had the chance to try it and get to appreciate its undoubted pleasures. What used for a while to be regarded as a low-down trick of some French prostitutes has at last found its way into the respectable bedrooms of western society.

For oral sex the penis should be clean. It should have been washed but not too recently. Twice daily washing with ordinary soap and water is enough. This means that just enough smegma will collect to produce a slight aroma. (Even in the circumcised there is a little about). Strangely, some men are put off by the penis smell, but most women are affected by it although they may not notice. It contains powerful aromatic chemicals that have the same, often subconscious, effect as does the scent of flowers to insects. Tiny traces can attract them. Careful medical tests have shown that women react similarly even in non-sexual situations, when minute penis aromas are released into the room. Things like blood pressure, respiration rate, pupil dilation, and even spontaneous uterine and vaginal contractions take place. The woman is being turned on without knowing it. This is one of the reasons why women so quickly become accustomed to sucking the penis.

The things that we call turn-ons are in effect release mechanisms. A woman may not be excited by the actual sight and touch of the penis or by having it in her mouth, but at the very least she is likely to undergo some stimulation from its scent. Oral sex quickly becomes part of the sex pattern. The same exactly is true of the vulva and vagina for the male.

The ways in which the penis can be treated by the mouth have no limit. The lips brushing it, the knob gently nibbled, the shaft stroked by the lips. The testicles can be softly sucked into the mouth singly or both together if the mouth is big enough. There is no way to tell a woman how to do it. She will soon develop her own style. She may slide the knob into one cheek, or holding it in her hand use it to 'brush her teeth.' She may tongue it all over or force the stiffened tip of her tongue into its opening. She may suck on it, quite hard. But she must never blow into it. The Americanism for having the penis sucked is a 'blow job.' It is very misleading. Air can be blown right back into the bladder or further. It hurts and it can be dangerous. Don't do it.

Some women are able to take a penis right past the mouth and well down into the throat, an action known as deep-throating. Linda Lovelace made a famous film about it. In the film the heroine's clitoris is far down her throat. That's only a story and is, of course, impossible. But the ability to accept the penis by relaxing the throat muscles so that it can be put in to the hilt is certainly possible. It is a technique to learn slowly and patiently. The rewards are worth it and problems virtually non-existent. But he should bear one thing in mind. Something touching the back of the throat makes one gag or even vomit. That can happen when a penis touches parts of a girl's throat. She can't help it. When she retches its not because she hates his penis but because it touched the wrong spot. Don't be too eager until you've both learned how.

And what about ejaculating into the mouth and throat? It might be worth reading over again the chapter about semen. Quite literally this time it's largely a matter of taste. Although the main constituents of semen don't alter, subtle differences of content can result from some foods eaten in the last day or two. Also the flavour of a woman's mouth varies with what else has recently been in it. So the same man's semen may not always taste the same. Some women are not happy about sucking a man off unless they can also have his semen. They love to swallow it. Others differ. In the latter case the penis can be withdrawn at the last moment and the ejaculation can be over her breasts and face or into a hand or handkerchief. (Oriental women massage it in as a facial cosmetic for which it is highly prized. I have also heard from European women that doing this daily for two weeks definitely improves the complexion. They were very convinced but I have no way of confirming this).

Three things are sure. If you like it you can do it as often as you like. There is absolutely no harm in swallowing semen. You cannot in any way get pregnant from an oral sex episode whether he ejaculates of not.

**Anal sex**
WARNING: This section is specifically for readers in regions where anal sex is legal; nothing written here should be interpreted as encouraging or even condoning any form of illegal activity.

In some places anal sex is illegal, for example, in several of the United States. Furthermore, until quite recent years in England a man could have it with another man but not with his wife whether she wants it or not. In spite of legal sanctions, like most enjoyable things, people do it just the same. And for those who like anal sex it can be very good indeed. I occasionally get patients of both sexes who come because they are worried about the whole thing. The essential is to reassure them that lots of people do it, perhaps even most people try it now and again. There is nothing abnormal about it. She may get very intense sensations. He finds the tight grip of the anus very pleasurable. The enjoyment doesn't mean that he is becoming homosexual or that she is perverted.

Anal intercourse is very common, but it is often unsuccessful and this is probably why it tends to be an occasional thing only. To enjoy it there are two essentials. First both must overcome any mental blocks that it is dirty or not nice in some way. Second, the anus is not primarily designed for intercourse, just as the lungs are not designed for smoking and human feet are not designed for sliding down mountains. The anus needs preparation if it is to be used for other than its original purpose. After training there is no reason why the female anus should not accept an average, full-sized and fully erected penis. The female anus is, after all, anatomically identical with the male anus,.. and homosexuals have little trouble training the orifice for sexual purpose.

No one is able to train her anus as well as the woman herself. Starting with a soapy finger in the bath perhaps, she gets the orifice used to accepting the intrusion. It is as well to look for specially pleasurable sensitive spots; these abound in both the anus and the vagina. After a while two fingers can be pushed in and eventually the tips of three. There are surgical instruments (e.g. Lord's dilator) designed for the purpose but a decent vibrator as long as it is thick enough is just as useful. Dilating the anus this way for five minutes a day is adequate over the course of a week or two to prepare it for sexual intercourse. Many users find the sensations so rewarding that they subsequently use the anus too for masturbatory pleasures.

There are as many variations for anal penetration as for vaginal but generally speaking three are most used; with her laying face down, kneeling, or on her back. Face down is the best one to start with. If the surface is firm she cannot pull away from the penetrating penis, and even if she is very keen, there comes a moment when, until she is used to it, she may try. Also, face down the buttocks prevent too deep penetration by the male beginner.

Before inserting the penis it is better if he or she puts a finger or two in during the love-play. At the selected moment and with plenty of lubricant on the penis and the anus, he should grasp the glans and compress it between his fingers and thumb. Thus reduced in size the glans is pushed against the orifice so that the same finger and thumb are at the anal margin. In this way they guide the penis in the right direction. Her response is to 'bear down' as if she were going to open her bowels. This relaxes the sphincter muscle that closes the orifice and the knob should enter easily. For a few seconds the penis is left quite still, just inside the orifice, as the muscle tends reflexly to contract. It soon relaxes again more thoroughly. Only then should the shaft of the penis be pushed further in, slowly and gently, allowing time for the orifice to accommodate it.

The technique for kneeling penetration is identical but when it comes to her lying on her back there is an extra tip. She needs a pillow under her hips and to have her thighs drawn well up and apart. He should kneel well astride so that he can lower his angle of approach. The penis should be about parallel with the bed. Once he is in he can lie on her as for vaginal intercourse. She will usually prefer this position because of the clitoral friction accompanying it. He needs care not to penetrate too deeply too soon.

There are no special problems with anal intercourse that training and lubrication will not obviate. However, infection, although rare, must be guarded against. Bacteria live in the rectum without harm. Transferred elsewhere they can be a nuisance. Always wash well before and after, not forgetting to scrub the fingernails. Never put anything, including the penis, into the vagina after it has been in the anus, without washing it first. Bacteria can be kept out of the male urethra by wearing a condom. Care needs to be taken that the tighter sphincter does not tear the sheath and that this is of a type suitable for use with a lubricant if that is the intention. Another good routine is to drink a pint of water half an hour before intercourse and urinate straight afterwards. Healthy urine is sterile and rinses out the urethra.

Anal intercourse can be a great pleasure for both partners. It is not suitable for rare use. Only the individual couple can decide how much they want it and whether the effort of training it is justified.

**Transvestism and transsexualism**

Although these are grouped together for convenience, they are not the same thing or even necessarily different degrees of the same thing. The transsexual feels that he or she lives in a body of the wrong sex, and is mentally and physically unsuited and perhaps unable to support life in the sexual role in which cast. There is a deep and genuine desire to assume the role of the opposite sex and extreme lengths may be gone to achieve this aim. It is a medical problem worthy of great sympathy and care. So-called sex change surgery may be indicated. The unfortunate woman may otherwise attempt to sew up her vulva or even attach an artificial penis. The man may actually attempt to castrate himself or sever the entire penis if he cannot get anyone else to do it for him. We see a substantial number of the more moderate degree of cases among women but more extreme cases among men.

The transvestite on the other hand is someone who merely gets pleasure from wearing clothes of the opposite sex. This may be simply restricted to during sexual intercourse or may involve other times too. More men are involved than women. The first thing that she must understand, if he is a transvestite, is that he is not any the less male for it. He does not feel female, he is not homosexual and he does not wish in anyway, including sexual, to exchange real roles, or identify as a female. It is a particularly difficult barrier for her to cross that her man wants to dress up in bra and panties. If she realises that in some way we do not understand it acts as a huge anxiety-reducing trick she will see it in its true light.

Transvestism is closely associated with fetishism which is also much more common in men than in women. It may range from a teenager wearing a stolen pair of his sister's panties to masturbate into, to the adult man who wants to dress from the skin out in women's wear. For the transvestite, wearing women's clothing is a highly exciting and rewarding sexual activity. It is well worth acting out if it's what he likes,.. and she can go along with it. Curiously, although quite large number of women have difficulty enjoying sex when their partners are dressed as women, men, when faced with transvestite wives, are more easily able to help act out the fantasy.

**Sadomasochism**

Sado-masochism (SM) is a vast field of sexual deviation which is sometimes carried to the vilest extremes of perversion. It is really comprised of two components which may be present together or may be separately manifested. Sadism is getting a kick out of hurting someone else. Masochism is getting a kick out of someone hurting you or you hurting yourself. Spanking, whipping, chaining, and tying up all belong in the sphere of SM/Bondage/Flagellation. [Jokes abound. For example there was the masochist who liked to take a cold bath in the morning,... so he took a hot one. Or, the difference between them, a masochist says, "Please hurt me" and the sadist replies, "No."]

No can adequately explain why pain has such a close association with pleasure. Very often the things that are pleasant in small amounts would be dangerous if carried too far. Examples of this are that plenty of people enjoy getting or giving a spanking. A severe hiding would be different. Some of the nerves that supply the genital area are also involved with skin surfaces notably over the buttocks and thighs. Being spanked on those surfaces can cause erection and intense sexual excitement in male and female. The value of spanking in encouraging desire and in treating impotence has been well known for centuries. Catherine the Great of Russia is reputed to have had attractive servants of both sexes on the payroll whose job it was to chastise the royal backside and thus encourage re-arousal when the Empress was exhausted by her notorious sexual excesses.

The stretching of the body sphincters may hurt and be pleasant at the same time. The pain/pleasure of emptying the bowels of large motions is well known. In describing their pleasures in sex many women will highlight the thrilling ecstasy of the moment of penetration of one or other orifice and its sphincter. The descriptions of their loss of virginity may also contain references to the "sweet pain," of the first dilatation of the vaginal sphincter.

Other factors may be at work especially in bondage and flagellation scenes. Some psychological explanations are obvious. There is a sensation of power and domination over a bound partner that is likely to be totally absent from all other aspects of life. But deeper motivations may be present. A childhood remnant of parent-dependence, perhaps from an environment of firm (and thus safe, predictable) discipline is frequently found. The matching of the fear of misuse while bound against the confident certainty that injury will not result offers a sensation of excitement similar, some think, to betting on horses or taking part in dangerous sports. A child, playfully cuffed on the ear, will gurgle with pleasure and return time and again for another cuff.

This is not the place for a detailed description of SM activities except for those that directly concern the penis. There is an unfortunate group of men who only get sexual pleasure from humiliation. At its most harmless this takes the form of having the partner act the part of the severe mistress while the 'slave', dressed perhaps as a housemaid, performs menial tasks about the house and is as a small reward, allowed to kiss the mistress' feet or get to intercourse, or actually be spurned and deliberately disappointed at the end. Believe it or not, that adds to the fun. At the other end of the scale the practice is again carried to dangerous extremes. A great favourite is to trap the root of the penis and testicles in some way so that pressure can be exerted gradually and excruciatingly until the pain becomes unbearable. Getting a partner to bite the penis or literally draw blood by lacerating the scrotum with stiletto heels are only some of the brutalities to which the penis is submitted. Expensive torture parlours exist in many cities. One can only offer one piece of advice to men who want to be mutilated in this way. Don't do it! Sadly, the advice will most certainly not be heeded.

**Sex crime**
Most, if not all, sex crime is the product of poor law and ignorant society. The more religious and [sexually] repressive an upbringing is, the greater the risk of moral deviancy and sexual violence later in life. This author's opinion is that, in fact, sex crime hardly exists. What people *call* sex crime certainly does, but the definition is questionable. Largely, the infringements that do occur are either so trivial as to be unworthy of their classification as crime, or, by their very nature are not really sexual. For example there is the very real crime of rape; this however, is not actually a sex crime but is a crime of violence with sex used as the weapon.

There is no more logical reason why a man should show his face to a strange woman than he should show his penis. It is we who have declared revealing the penis something offensive. If a woman accidentally chances upon an undressed man invariably his penis will attract the larger share of her attention,... though she may deny this. The offence is in actually showing it to her, not in the penis itself. Men who exhibit themselves, the so-called 'flashers,' makers of dirty phone calls, and those who jostle and fumble against women in the subway [frottage] are inadequate, little maladjusted creeps taking an unmanly and unfair advantage. Usually the look of horror on the frightened woman's face is the kick. If women were not suitably shocked the whole thing would be pointless.

A few tips for the girls on how to deal with unwanted gentlemen, for example, the frotteur who deliberately rubs against you in the bus. If you don't care to enjoy it, (and some do) wait until the bus lurches, then crush your heel back onto his toe or your umbrella into his crotch. Better still, if you have the nerve, say at the top of your voice, "Why don't you take your hands off my arse and put them on his?" meanwhile nodding towards the biggest bloke you can see. Repeated phone calls are dealt with by keeping a referee's whistle near the phone. A fierce blast straight down the mouthpiece should raise blisters on his ear drums. Best of all was the accomplished business woman of my acquaintance who was accosted by a lad who flashed his limp penis at her in the underground. She looked at it with great concern and said, "Do be careful that horrid, limp little thing doesn't catch cold!"

**Masturbation**
This is only included here for convenience. There is nothing sinister about its appearance in this section of sexual variations except that it does provide the most useful and most widely used variation in, or substitute for, real sex that there is. Masturbation is an excellent thing. There is virtually nothing that can be said against it for either men or women, boys or girls. Until around the 1930s there was a concept, contributed to, I'm sorry to say, by doctors, educationalists and the clergy, that masturbation could lead to all kinds of dreadful conditions, blindness, weakness and serious physical, moral and mental deterioration. Men strapped their sons into mechanical devices that made masturbation impossible to preserve their moral purity.

Masturbation is to be encouraged for anyone who fancies it, and should have all associations of shame and guilt removed even for those who don't. Its value is five-fold. First, it is good practice,... for youngsters learning about sex or for older men, many of whom can still do with plenty of practice, it offers a way of learning how to control the approach to orgasm. A man can increase and decrease the excitement level so that on other occasions, when involved in the real thing, he is more skilled. This helps make his technique good and his timing precise. It also affords a measure of protection against sexual problems like premature ejaculation and impotence.

Second, it is a substitute. Many men are without sexual contact with a partner for a variety of reasons. They may live and work where there are no women,.. in the services or on contract jobs abroad. Their wives may be physically unfit for actual intercourse. Little, unattractive, poor, old and timid men can have great difficulty finding a partner with whom to satisfy their sex drive. Yet, it is vital to recognise, their sex drive is quite as powerful as that of the virile, wealthy, handsome giant. Perhaps it was the careful hand of nature, recognising the risks of perpetual frustration, that provided the substitute of masturbation. I have met vast numbers of men who have lived (and died) without having any other sexual outlet.

Third, even within a marriage there arise times when for one reason or another one partner needs more sexual activity than the other. Up to a point they can adjust and compensate, but the extent to which this succeeds is limited. Recourse to the use of masturbation restores the balance for however long it is needed.

Fourth, of all ways of learning about one's own and one's partner's sexual preferences, the best is with the use of masturbation. She should watch him. See where he holds himself, with finger and thumb or with his full fist. What angle does he use? How fast does he rub, and how tightly or loosely? He should watch her too. Does she rub her clitoris, or stroke her labia? Does she put anything in her vagina? How many fingers? How hard, how fast, and so on? Try talking during masturbation. When people masturbate they fantasise. Very few masturbate without fantasising; some experts believe it is probably not even possible. In their minds people create wild flights of imagination. They may imagine where they are, what they are doing or having done to them, the people with whom they are doing it. Some fantasies are far too secret to be discussed without shame or without hurting the other half, or risking being misunderstood. But many can be shared and just before orgasm (whether by intercourse or masturbation) is a good time. If you have not tried to learn more of your heart's desires by noticing carefully your fantasy sequences, then it's time you did. And if you are in a worthwhile relationship and have not yet agreed to this kind of communication, it is high time you did. Nothing will tell you more about yourself and your partner. Nothing provides a better foundation for a deep communication and understanding.

The fifth and last value of masturbation is that it is sexually exciting; it is nice. Of course it goes without saying that it is exciting to do it to yourself. It may also be a great turn-on to do it to your partner. And never forget how exciting it can be to others if not to you, to watch someone masturbate. If your partner enjoys watching you, let yourself go and offer a treat; and by all means anticipate the same in return.

There are as many techniques of masturbation as there are people to carry them out. So there are no useful instructions. But there are some useful tips. There's no harm in it, so do it as much as you like. Few people run at their best (although they may not admit or even know it) without two or three orgasms a week. Make sure your hands are clean, especially of things like detergents, garden sprays and the like. Don't be dismayed if his ejaculate [if any] is less second time than the first; it invariably is. Don't be surprised if her second orgasm is more powerful than her first, it often is. Don't regard masturbation as an alternative for real sex except where real sex is unavailable. It is an extra, not a substitute.

\* \* \*

The problem for all of us, when we come across a new sexual phenomenon, is not to be put off by it. No-one must react automatically if they can help it. Reacting is thoughtless; thinking is far better. See your own and your partner's pet fancies for what they are, a part of his or her developing personality. If you don't like that personality you have no business being there. Sexual preferences or deviations are not diseases. They are the present result of years of complex interacting influences. They are expanding, developing,... varying all the time, and always will be.

You are lucky to have the chance of sexual variety,... go ahead and enjoy it.

\* \* \* \* \*

# SECTION TWO:
# THE PENIS AROUND THE WORLD
**Chapter Six:** The Penis in Art
## Sexual suppression

In view of the monumental importance of the penis, it comes as nothing of a surprise to find that it has featured very prominently in the entire field of art. From the earliest times right up to modern days it can be found making a significant contribution in every branch and facet of the artistic world. In painting, drawing, sculpture and literature there are gems of inspiration and expression which stem from relevance of the penis in particular and sex in general. No aspect has been excluded. What has been lacking has been exposure,.. in this context meaning the tolerance and permission to display erotic art publicly.

Of course if you subject entire growing populations, from infancy, to the concept that sex is dirty, evil and forbidden, they will grow up accepting that concept as truth. With education and the onset of reason, later on some will reject the nonsense. Many never will and others will be afraid to say they've changed their minds. Such unenlightened folk continue to be offended and frightened by published sexual material. In a democratic society, these deprived folk are nevertheless deemed to be in need of protection. The only way to achieve that is for all people to be subjected to restrictions, by censorship if necessary, and prevented from enjoying sexual material.

In most of the world's great religions there are cautions about sex and its effects. Rarely if ever though, are there any serious curtailments of the enjoyment of sex and sexual activities. Certainly there is little in the teachings, for example, of Jesus of Nazareth, that could be regarded as draconian in sexual matters.

Despite this, the sick and distorted minds that were loaded with the immense responsibility of teaching the new and gentle religion of Christianity to a largely pagan world saw fit, by some bizarre and perverse corruption of logic, to suppress or curb sexuality. This all fitted in quite well with the fundamental principles of Judaism, and later, Christianity, both of which rely heavily upon concepts of human sin, remorse, humiliation and general unworthiness. Perhaps it was felt that anything as enjoyable as sex simply had to be a bad thing. But whatever the confused logic used, the result was that anything even mildly erotic was ruthlessly extirpated. Before the advent of Christianity there is little evidence to show that many people connected the idea of sex with the idea of being 'dirty.' Sex was hitherto a natural and accepted process as capable of being involved in art and literature as the sun, moon and the flowers. Suppression has never been more than partly successful.

It can be accepted that religion is a fountainhead of artistic inspiration. In the same way, as sex is of greater fundamental importance to more men than is religion, so sex is at least as great a source of artistic inspiration,.. but only if allowed to be.

Happily, the level of suppression is falling as the concepts of Christianity recede before the pressures of the changing world. The magnificent, tender sculpture of white marble that is Rodin's 'The Kiss' was classed as pornographic when first completed. Now it stands in the Tate Gallery and pictures of it have even adorned the London Underground. Good sense triumphs, if slowly. A shining example of this was in the late sixties when the internationally famous Kronhausens staged an Exhibition of Erotic Art in Sweden and Denmark,.. but more of that later.

**The primitive penis**

Amongst the earliest paintings and sculptures found in caves in France and the Sahara and dating from Neolithic times sex is prominently represented. Amongst primitive sculptured figures from the ruins of Mesopotamia and the round-house dwellings of prehistoric man, already the penis was a favoured feature. Even in England near the quiet Dorset town of Cerne Abbas is what must surely be the largest penis if not in the entire world, then at least in the British Isles. Standing erect and naked and every inch of thirty feet long it is the property of the giant figure cut through the turf into the chalk layer of a nearby hillside. No one knows who shaped the Cerne Abbas Giant, or why, or how many hundreds or more likely thousands of years ago he was hewn. But his penis is vast. Hugely erected and standing up tight against his abdomen, the penis has two superbly shaped testicles precisely proportioned and realistically suspended with one a little larger and hanging a little lower down than the other.

Prehistoric paintings show men and animals copulating as well as women and animals. Monstrous, stylised penises (penes) sprout from humans, animals, and even tree trunks. In some cases they were probably fertility symbols or portrayals of actual fertility rites. Others are examples of the parallel magic whereby in some way the picturing of an act or an object influenced the happenings in the picture to take place in reality. Some examples, perhaps are just the wishful thinking of the artist and bear only the same relation to truth as does the vast bulging graffiti penis drawn on the door of any public toilet in modern day London.

**The sophisticated penis**

The Indian subcontinent has enjoyed a high level of civilisation throughout long periods of its history. It is in such situations that art flourishes. The sexual art of India is therefore second to none. Famous amongst that art is the huge array of figures carved into the living rock of some temples. Temples were regarded as fitting places for such sculpture and the Black Pagoda of Konarak, some two hundred and fifty miles from Calcutta, is singularly memorable. Countless men, women and animals writhe around each other stroking, sucking and copulating in a contortion of limbs and bodies and practising among them a tableaux of every imaginable, deviant sexual variation.

Less free in style was the rigid interpretation of art that came with the civilisation of Egypt. Apart from ribald graffiti there is little sexual art anyway. What there is is in the classical poses of Pharaonic carving. The one noticeable thing is that if a man's penis is shown, it is invariably longer or thicker than in real life and is shown standing up at a superb angle. Regrettably, a primitive Christian sect once lived in the old, crumbling temples of the Nile. These, mostly Copts, were guilty amongst other things of building fires against irreplaceable carved figures, of using tombs as repositories of their excrement and refuse, and of defacing many of the figures, particularly their heads, breasts, and the genital organs. Enlightenment and religious dedication are not always found together.

Of all the western world's known great ancient sources of erotic art, pride of place must go without question to Pompeii. This flourishing Roman town was buried by falling ashes from the erupting Vesuvius one midsummer night in the year 79 AD. The thriving and sophisticated city afterwards lay almost untouched until the Eighteenth Century. Then intrepid excavators and profiteers began searching the ruins. To their astonishment a remarkably rich source of erotic material was uncovered. Much of it was dedicated to characterisations of the human penis. So offensive was the material to prudish eyes that it was mostly stored in a secret room in a Naples museum. A larger collection of erotica even than that belonging to the Vatican was assembled. It was strictly private until the decision in 1973 of the new director, Professor Alfonso de Franciscis, to open it to the public. At last the huge phallic statues, books, and pictures were available to everyone.

One of the most remarkable pictures in Pompeii is a wall painting in the House of the Vetii. These wealthy brothers were wine merchants and much given to the pursuit of happiness, which inevitably included the happiness of pursuit. Their most famous picture is of a character known as *Il Commandante*, (The Commander). In his portrait he stands next to a weighing scales. His vast penis hangs in one tray while the other tray is laden with gold and gems. Indeed one famous visiting lady is reputed to have looked and commented, "Now that's what I call a 14-carat jewel." I was unable to find out for certain which tray she was looking at.

The Commander is not alone however. In the secret room there are literally hundreds of vases, pictures, mosaics, amulets, plates and lamps, the fine artwork of which is overtly sexual in its nature. Not surprisingly, the penis, often depicted as vastly larger than life size, is widely exploited as a subject, and not only in the artwork. For tucked away in the brickwork of Pompeii's excavated streets are special signs pointing the way to the Lupanare, the brothel. The signs are specially designed bricks, not with a pointing arrow or finger, but with a large erect penis pointing the way. The intention is perfectly clear,.. and not in the least outdated.

Some architecture may not be without a sexual association. Is it, for example, a pure coincidence that so many kinds of monuments have taken the form of a tall slender shape rising from the ground? Is it possible, as has been suggested, that obelisks like Cleopatra's Needle, towers, and even church spires and steeples are inspired by the deep emotional significance of the erect penis? Certainly the shape is unmistakable. In more ancient times the huge monoliths, single standing stones, were even less disguised. Some people are so familiar with this form of structure that they have come to regard it as a naturally occurring building form. There is, of course, no such thing. All of man's ideas, however obvious, sprang from some inspirational source. The theory may be confused and exaggerated but it has the ring of truth and I, for one, would not dismiss it out of hand. And what natural shape inspired the favoured domes of Rome, the Moslem world and St. Paul's Cathedral, many of them adorned with a small extra projection at their summit? The resemblance to breasts and nipples is almost too obvious to be ignored.

**The liberated penis**

When we come to consider the most abundant kind of art, pictorially displayed drawings, paintings, etchings and so on, it is here that sexual expression reaches a summit. Some sexual art is very old. Some is very modern. But what is very modern indeed, at least in relation to the last couple of hundred years is the displaying of sexual art. Under the crippling fetters of hypocritical and misled religious thought, sex was equated with evil and its expression was discouraged or frankly forbidden. In recent decades we have seen the false foundations of the edifice of alleged obscene material shaken and largely demolished. Twenty years ago even a 'respectable' nudist magazines was not allowed to show pubic hair. It was as if it were too disgusting or evil or didn't exist. Now gradually, and with a fierce battle for every step, it has become possible to show at least some phenomena the way they are. The Scandinavian countries have been the world's leaders in this direction and no one more so than the Kronhausens. This husband and wife team wrote a book, Erotic Art, on the exhibition thereof that they organised in 1968. This subtle, sensitive, humorous and exciting collection thrilled thousands of international visitors. If it did one thing useful it was to strip a lot of foolish mystique from the subject. Children were not terrified by it after all, and no one gave vent to the predicted attacks of sexual frenzy. Above all no one had to watch. They didn't have to come in at all and if they did they could just as easily leave.

One of the oldest objects on display was a grotesque little terra-cotta man from the Mexico of 400 BC. It is a seated figure with a huge phallus similar to the phallic statutes of other parts of the world or the Pompeiian Commander. There was also a clever and intricately designed decoration from ancient Peru. A man and woman of silver uncouple and recouple in a variety of positions. Old Indian pictures show men putting the penis up through the hole in the floorboards to enjoy a lady while her husband sits reading to her. Another popular Indian theme is of competitions, much like the Knobbly Knees contests of today's village fetes, but where the competition is for the largest, ugliest penis. Some ingenious methods of measuring have been tried.

The Japanese contributions are much concerned with what always appears to be an Eastern obsession with penis size. Sigimura Jihei (17th century) shows girls, their toes curled in the abandon of their passions, with vast penises assaulting their wide-open genitalia. From the 18th century, Ohyo, a famous painter of Kyoto naturalism, shows male members of anything but natural size, shape and colour. They are brown, warty and thicker by far than a human wrist. The only thing about them that strikes one as natural is the degree of delight they appear to afford penetrator and penetrated alike. Also, it appears, none of today's so-called advanced sexual techniques seem to be all that new. Yamato delicately displayed two friends enjoying opposite ends of the same girl in the 18th century and Moroshiga was fond of showing a couple watching their own intercourse in a carefully placed mirror.

The Chinese, on the other hand, seem less concerned with penis size than with technology. Funniest by far is a picture of a couple each hung in a cloth cradle from the branches of neighbouring trees. Their servants are swinging them together hopefully to meet with a comforting measure of accuracy in the centre.

More up-to-date, there is a free indulgence in sexual expressionism. 'Le Pianotaur,' a musical instrument turned animal, copulates with a woman in a picture by Andre Masson. From Austria in 1910 came Franz Von Bayros' delicate engraving of two young girls playing and dildoing themselves in a huge ornate and mirrored bed. Hans Bellmer's superb erotic drawings reach magnificent heights of imagination. In them masturbating fingers merge anatomically into vulva or anus, penises into sucking mouths and genitalia male and female into each other in a pictorial display of the capacity of sexual contact so real that it transcends any verbal description. Even more modern is the work of the contemporary American erotic artist, Betty Dodson, with her voluptuous locked and intertwined couples, the subtle eroticism of Italian Stanislav Lepri, and the overwhelming blatant sexual exhibitionism of Cesare Peverelli.

The market for pornography or 'dirty pictures' throughout the world remains enormous. Because in some countries it is still suppressed, it has become a commodity of the Black Market, and is now irrevocably linked to organised crime. Its cost has become extortionate. A few enlightened countries, Denmark, Sweden, and Holland were the first, abolished their anti-pornography laws. They did not suffer the predicted horrors of increased sex crime.

A Royal Commission in UK and a Congressional Committee in USA pronounced in favour of permitting a considerable amount of pornographic material to be circulated. Nonetheless, confusion and religious fundamentalism continued the illogical suppression. Much pornography is dull, repetitive and banal. Some is brilliant, beautiful, erotic and instructive,.. for example the magnificent work of Swedish photographer-publisher Berth Milton,.. a valued personal friend of this author. Regrettably, almost all of his work remains banned in Great Britain and the United States, though more enlightened European countries are pleased to allow and enjoy it.

At eighteen you can marry and vote. You can be entrusted with fighting,.. and dying, for your country. But you cannot be entrusted with sexy pictures!!

How's that for logic?

**The humorous penis**

One particular item from the above mentioned Kronhausen Exhibition brings us to our next subject. It was a humorous one. It was a latex rubber cushion from which, at exactly the correct angle, was moulded a shapely erect penis. The cushion was on a firm chair and was listed as available 'for lonely ladies.' Sex and everything to do with it is one of the great sources of humour. Sometimes it is overtly male chauvinistic in origin. Other times it can applaud the penis and its prowess or, just as easily mock it, its appearance, ability and size. Nowhere is this seen more than in limericks. For example:

> There was a young fellow named Bliss
> Whose love-life was sadly amiss
> For even with Venus
> His recalcitrant penis
> Could never do better than t
>                               h
>                               i
>                               s.

Another example concerns the myth, remarkably widely known and even today half-believed, especially in the armed forces, that Chinese women have their genital orifice in the form of a side to side slit as opposed to the fore and aft anatomy of their western sisters. It is, of course, not so,.. as the limerick tells:

> A marine being sent to Hong Kong
> Got the doctor to alter his dong.
> He sailed off with a tool
> Thin and flat as a rule,
> But he got there and found he was wrong.

In addition to limericks, penis jokes abound. Take for the example the story of the fat, ugly, junior nurse instructed to go and shave a patient's penis before surgery. She surprised the senior nurse, a pretty and shapely girl, by explaining afterwards that she had been interested to find that the patient had the word 'Ludo' tattooed on his penis. Intrigued, the senior went to see for herself. Three quarters of an hour later she returned, looking a little dishevelled, and informed the nurse that the patient was a Welshman and the word was not Ludo but Llandudno!

Not every penis does as well. One well-known writer sardonically and cruelly described an impotent penis which was soft as a doughnut as the kind 'that was always hanging around with no visible means of support,.. soft as a marshmallow. And as he and she well knew, you can't squeeze a marshmallow into a moneybox.'

Without any semitic prejudice there seems no harm in observing that inference that Jews are the world's most conceited (or optimistic) people,.. they cut a bit off it even before they know how long its going to be.

And there is the famous quote embodying the alleged difference between the sexes,...

> Hogamus, higamus,
> Man is polygamous.
> Higamus, hogamus,
> Woman monogamous.

## The literary penis

One of the wittier comments in literature comes from the pen of Dahlberg who, in his book 'The Sorrows of Priapus' says, "... the entire tribe of pudenda and scroti have the heads of pygmies, and the wrinkles of stupidity, decrepitude and mirth." He goes on to liken the penis to an independent creature loaned and stuck onto a man. Once there it goes its own way as it chooses, dragging its perhaps reluctant owner with it. It may want to urinate when its owner wants to think, or to go to bed when he wants to read. Even worse, the owner may want to go and do a kindness to an old lady crossing the road but the tyrant penis wants to ejaculate because some shapely-bottomed girl just stooped over to pick up the laundry!

Sadly, even this harmless and amusing little morsel is known to all too few people as it fell foul of the dictates of the law. So much of literature, especially in the United Kingdom (that champion of freedom of speech, religion, and so on), has been kept from the eyes of its people. Until the 1970s The Banned Books of England filled four boxes of catalogue cards in the British (Museum) Library. Not only trivial, soft-core pornography,.. the Hank Janson and Raymond Chandler novels of the Forties and Fifties languish there, but for many decades so did some great literary works. Petronius' great classic Satyricon described Roman scenes of flagellation, fellatio, sodomy and the deflowering of little girls. No one would ban it today. After Boccaccio wrote his Decameron it was available to all to read. It was not placed in the Pope's forbidden list (the ludicrous and infamous Index Librorum Prohibitorum) until the next century. Even then it was so classified not because of its indecency but because of its blasphemy. Yet, five centuries later it remained banned in the UK. and the USA!

This is one of the problems about sexual material. It changes with the time, the place, the social environment, and so on. For example, when Maurice Girodias of the Olympia Press first had the courage to publish Nabokov's Lolita, it was denounced by John Gordon in the Sunday Express. Don Leavy's Ginger Man was similarly misunderstood. So was 'The Story of O'. At the same time the Book of Leviticus was being read in churches though (see chapter 20, verse 13) it seriously recommends the execution of homosexuals! Those who set out to guard the morals of their peers are seldom as pure as they would like us to believe. Their confusion often obscures their logical judgements.

A shining example of this is to be seen in the so-called Private Case of the British Museum. You need a personal letter from the Director after satisfying him that you are a bona fide serious worker before you can see the things that are in the that case. And when you see it, what do you find? Torrid steaming magazines from Stockholm demonstrating the carnal knowledge of maidens by wild beasts? Seldom indeed. You find the amusing secret poems of one Robert Burns, 'The Merry Muses' which wouldn't be repeatable on Burns Night. You find Beaudelaire and Voltaire and the suppressed works of Lord Byron. You find that same 'Story of O' though you can buy it openly in the Strand. You find photograph books with the pubic hair of men and women painted out and with the official stamp of a royal crown and the words 'British Museum' on the backs of all stealable photographs usually carefully positioned precisely behind the 'dirty' bits. Many of the books are in French, Spanish. Russian and German. Some date to the 1600's. There is even a book on the priapic treasures of the Naples National Museum we mentioned earlier. It is harmless and mostly rubbish. It gives the impression that it has not been looked at with any care for years.

This odd attitude has been noted and commented on by less confused foreign scholars many times. For example, writing his treatise on sex life in England in 1934, Dr. Iwan Bloch made a study and analysis of some of the foremost erotic and allegedly obscene classics. His conclusion was that they had a four-fold appeal, "... to the psychologist and psychoanalyst; to the literary critic, historian, philologist and bibliographer; to the fields of medical science, pathology, law and jurisprudence, and lastly, to the entire world of art which has been for so long bereft of the greatest erotic classics of English art and genius."

No-one I have ever heard of has come up with a valid objection to erotographic or even pornographic material. For pornography is never bad or harmful. At best it may be highly erotic and evocative, even artistically enthralling, expressive and beautiful. At the very worst, it is nothing more than trivial and boring. Repeated attempts have been made to connect pornography with evidence of it being able to induce crime and anti-social sexual behaviour. Every reliable assessment so far has failed to do this. Reactionary influences have tried to associate the sex and violence as if they were inseparable. In fact they are not so. Indeed, they overlap about as much as do law and justice, which is to say, not a great deal.

Happily, in spite of the misguided, if at least sometimes genuine, efforts at suppression, art of all types continues to recognise sex and all matters sexual as an abundant source and a justifiable means of artistic interpretation and expression. Sex in its way is an art. And there is little that can be more capable of artistic portrayal than the human body,.. including its phallus.

\* \* \* \* \*

**Chapter Seven:** Myths and Legends

It is entirely fitting that a subject that has been one of the great motivating influences of all time should also have been the source of a vast compendium of legend and mythology. Sadly, as with so many myths, many of those that surround the penis and its sexual prowess are mere nonsense. There is, for example, a story that suggests a connection between the size of a man's nose and the size of his penis. This particular myth dies hard, although there is not a shred of truth in it. It is particularly widely believed amongst women. As a result, it appears many a woman has conducted a studied chase of a man with a large nose only to be shattered with a great disappointment when she catches him.

**Racial penis envy**

In the Book of Enoch it tells that the world's first two-legged creatures, whoever they were, had large genitalia. Another tale about the big penis is that of its racial differences. If we are to believe the authorities of the period of slavery, especially in the Southern States of America, we will hear that the alleged great penis size of the black slaves was a constant, perceived threat to the whites. Knowing that their black male slaves were often equipped with penises larger than their own they came to fear that a white woman who had had a black man would never again want a white one. Much of the ferocity with which slavery was conducted resulted from this false fear. Even after slavery had been abolished, and indeed, to this very day, the horror and fear which is associated with miscegenation in America and South Africa is partly rooted in this particular aspect of unfavourable competition. The truth of the matter is pointed out by the able Indian expert Chakrovarti in his book on sex life in India. Although black African men do tend to have larger penises in the flaccid state, the extent of their enlargement and the degree of rigidity is no greater than for whites, if indeed quite as great. Some women do declare a preference for a less than rigid penis but these are few. It would thus appear that grounds for this spiteful fear between races are shaky indeed. Indian (brown) men tend to have longer but thinner penises than Europeans.

**The religious penis**

One of the earliest and most important myths to concern the penis takes place in the pantheistic hierarchy of the Nile Delta of Ancient Egypt. The great god-king Osiris is invited to a feast by his brother, Set. By treachery Osiris is done to death and cut into thirteen pieces, one for each lunar month. His consort goddess, Isis, hides from Set and gives birth to the hawk-god Horus, son of Osiris. Assisted by Horus' magic vision, Isis reassembles the body of her husband only to find that one piece, the penis, is missing,.. eaten by the fishes. Isis is reputed to have made a substitute symbol of the vital missing organ. So far it is mythology, but it is true that an image of the Osirian penis some fifty yards long was later carried by priests during the relevant religious festivals. The symbol may indeed have later given rise to the prominence of the obelisks and standing stones and pillars favoured in Egyptian architecture. Eventually, as the myth tells, Horus fights Set for supremacy and the other gods declare in Horus' favour but not before he, in his turn, has severed the penis of Set. This ritual emasculation is not without its significance and the practice of brutally removing the penis from every man dead, wounded or taken prisoner in battle survived sporadically for many centuries,.. and, if press reports are to be believed, has re-emerged in the last decade.

The penis of Set achieved greater significance in mythological history. Hidden, dried and passed from owner to owner, it, or whatever represented it, came to be recognised as a most powerful focus of evil. Known as the Talisman of Set, it has recurred time and again through the history of occultism even up to fairly recent popular writers in the field of necromancy and witchcraft (see Dennis Wheatley: *'The Devil Rides Out.'*)

The penis as a symbol naturally had values in fertility rites. In Roman times it was common to hang a phallic symbol, for example a *fascis*, or bundle, around the necks of babies. Some students of language have suggested that our own word to fascinate may be connected to this same potency sign; the connection between fascination and fertility may indeed not be totally absent.

'Unto the pure all things are pure: but unto them that are defiled and unbelieving is nothing pure; but even their mind and conscience is defiled.' So says the Bible (Titus 1 v. 15): I mention that quotation in order to avert criticism that may arise from my forthcoming comments on the Bible. For the Bible contains many things that could be regarded as impure by the defiled mind. I make no such allegation of impurity. The rape of Tamar by her brother (2. Samuel 13 v. 14) and the approbation given to the incest of Lot's daughters with their father, albeit for a good cause, (Genesis 10, v.30-36) draws, from this author, no comment! Nor even does the suggestion in Genesis 2 v.20 that Adam sought a mate amongst the available animal kingdom before Eve appeared on the scene.

However, a highly significant act concerning the penis is mentioned in the Bible and thus has its place here. This is the act of using the penis as the subject on which an oath of great importance might be sworn. Deference is paid to decorum by using an euphemistic alternative expression. Instead of directing that the hand of the oath-swearer be placed on his penis, as was in fact the custom, the phrase used concerns putting the hand 'under the thigh.' Abraham makes his senior servant swear in this way in Genesis 24 v.2. Later in Chapter 47 (v.29) Joseph also swears his oath in like manner. The penis, the most sacred part of a man's body, was suitable for the most significant and binding oaths. The idea is not altogether lost even now. In Wales in medieval times there was extant under the decree of King Hywel the Good, the law that a woman must publicly identify a man she accused of rape while placing her right hand on holy relics and her left hand simultaneously on the penis of the alleged rapist. There was to be no doubt. One can but ponder the likelihood of such an identity parade in today's criminal court proceedings!

The use of penis-shaped objects as well as shapes resembling female sexual organs has been well known in attempts to influence the degree of fertility. In ancient times fertility was everything. A strong nation, an expanding economy and even the support of a man in his later years rested ultimately on a continuous and steady increase in every commodity. First and foremost was the need for more and more people. Nothing was so great and so useful a sign of the certainty of the future as the fertility of one's fields, herds and most of all one's family. Any act that could propitiate gods into increasing fertility was vital. Any object that could influence the bountiful hand of nature was an advantage. Sexual objects were high on the list of tried and perceived as successful fertility-improving methods.

The vegetable kingdom has always provided phallic objects galore. They range from simple Maypoles to huge trees felled across sacred groves and then carved down roughly to resemble a penis before being danced on or decorated. At the other end of the scale, fruits like cucumbers and bananas have had their significance for obvious reasons.

Animals too provided such symbols often in the form of horns [of plenty] and also in the taunting of vicious male animal instincts as in cock fighting, bear baiting, and in the bull ring. Even geological formations have been used. Occasionally groups of people have attached importance to certain projecting portions of land vaguely penis-shaped and jutting out into sea or lake. Sailing a barren woman around these in a boat, usually for a certain mystical number of times, or on certain days or lunar phases, could make her fertile again.

There was a parallel to this phallic fertility symbolism on the female side too. A cleft in a rock resembled a vaginal cleft and might house a temple or church. (There is one such at St. Govan's in Dyfed in Wales today). Caves, like the magical cave of the oracle at Delphi in Ancient Greece or the famous grotto at Lourdes, had similar comparisons with the female sexual organ. Until recent times there was a large stone in the Cornish village of Mardon. Through it was a natural fourteen-inch hole and people were passed through this as a form of symbolic rebirth to try to cure them from certain ailments. Where no such naturally formed object existed, an artificial one was frequently created. A young ash tree would be split down its main stem and opened out like a vulva. Naked children were then symbolically reborn three times through the split tree being passed from female hand to male. The tree was afterwards bound up and as it healed (ash trees in particular heal very well in this way), the child's ailment was cured. This method was also used as a treatment for impotence. The ineffective penis was passed through the open tree stem while spells were spoken or herbal remedies applied. If conducted especially at propitious phases of the stars and planets, this magic ensured that the becalmed penis regained its potency.

The use of the priapus, or erect phallus, or at any rate some form of dildo, is also found in the coming of age ceremonies or sometimes the marriage ceremonies of some tribes. With some peoples a particular phallic replica of religious association was used. The reasoning behind it is confused but appears to be several-fold. The forceful rupture of the virgin's hymen with the god-phallus was likely to engender fertility. Furthermore, as the god thus had all virgins first, he would be pleased and propitiated; also as no men ever had a virgin first, no man would be made jealous of another in a community in which fighting between male adults was counter-productive. The savage way in which this first penetration was conducted caused great pain and profuse bleeding, thus demonstrating the virginity of the girl to one and all and ensuring that she brought honour to her family and her new husband alike. The act of deflowering was generally very thoroughly done, the initiation penis being of merciless size and brutal handling. This in turn meant that the girl was most adequately stretched to start with. She was thus forcibly introduced to and made accustomed to penetration. Her husband was spared the dubious and tedious delights of defloration, and all guilt or blame for the act was removed from him. She became sexually enjoyable without much further effort on his part and hopefully, the whole procedure avoided, for him, the continued dislike and nagging of his wife for any natural clumsiness he might have displayed when depriving her of her maidenhead.

With a typically complicated comment, the great student of the human mind, Carl Jung, warned that in his view the consideration of the penis as a symbol was not without its risks. His opinion was that with a phallic symbol the symbolism does not represent the phallus but rather, the libido, the vital urge of sexuality that activated the organ.

Since the oldest times the male symbol was not merely the penis but some ever-rutting, darkness-penetrating, activating and enriching entity. In dreams the penis is to be regarded as the symbol of self and it is notable that dreaming frequently of the penis is a characteristic which, in psychoanalysis, suggests someone of low sexuality.

Whereas the female by tradition is symbolically associated with maternal things, stillness, solidity, spontaneity, fruitfulness and one-ness, the male connects with matters of the spirit,... dynamic, volatile and productive. The male is represented, understandably, by things that are long and penetrating like the arrow, finger, sword and plough; things upright, like pillars and trees; things fiery, sun, light and heat; and things prolific and strong, the bull, the lion, and war.

**Drugs, potions and potency**

The last great myth of all perhaps that it seems almost a shame to have to demolish is the list of foods and other consumables that can make the penis perform better. Somewhere or other and at some time almost everything has been claimed to be aphrodisiac. Aphrodisiacs are declared by some to be non-existent, but are fondly believed to exist by many others. The fact is that aphrodisiacs do exist in that there are things which improve human sexual arousal, response, staying power, performance and pleasure. Detailed discussion is beyond the scope of this book and is far better covered elsewhere (see, for example, The Human Aphrodisiac by Dr. Steven Roles MD. See Bibliography).

The unfortunate thing is that many aphrodisiacs and substances have side-effects that are dangerous in doses that are likely to have any sexual effect. Spanish Fly (cantharides) is so dangerous that users could well be liable to charges of manslaughter in the event of mishap. Gold and silver salts, so popular with Asiatic populations, can cause heavy metal poisoning if only from the toxic contaminants like lead and tin that they contain. Ginseng can cause insomnia, diarrhoea and blood pressure. Alcohol works in small doses, as do pemoline and strychnine though poisoning by these is too likely to justify the risk.

Some foods are known to have aphrodisiac qualities as do some herbal preparations. A new technique is currently being developed and holds out perhaps the greatest possible hope of an effective aphrodisiac preparation at last being made commercially available.

A panel of doctors, pharmacists, herbalists and homoeopaths recently pooled their knowledge and experience. After scouring the extensive literature they selected the most successful known ingredients. Some of these are of recent discovery, others have been known for centuries. The component items have been processed for careful extraction of their active herbal contents. Once extracted they are subjected to radionic potentisation. This involves exposure in some of the most advanced equipment such as that produced by the famous De La Warr Laboratories, in Oxford, England. It is understood that they are now under final test as drops taken under the tongue or in small stimulant homoeopathic doses.

It is expected that they will combine efficiency as an aphrodisiac for men and women with the well known safety record of homoeopathic medicines. If they are made commercially available by the time this book goes to print, it is intended to mention them in the final appendix in the Sources List.

Regrettably, and in contrast to the real aphrodisiacs, few of the traditionally alleged aphrodisiacs actually work except perhaps psychologically. A little red pepper ground finely into butter and rubbed gently into the head of the penis and the vulval lips causes slight inflammation and a desire to rub, thereby somewhat increasing circulation, erection and engorgement. Some people enjoy this.

Some things are said to be aphrodisiac because they look like a penis. Asparagus is one such. Others represent a vulva, for example, half a peach. Chocolate is widely regarded as containing aphrodisiac components. It is this which has given rise to the tradition of offering gifts of chocolate on St.Valentine's Day. Shellfish are alleged to contain magically stimulating substances. Some of them do contain chemicals allied to animal sex hormones, though it is more likely that it is the appearance, flavour and texture of oysters wherein lies their aphrodisiac quality. Certainly eating and drinking together in sexually alert circumstances can exaggerate the sexual feelings and improve performance afterwards. It is the atmosphere that produces the majority of the effect, even if the physical acts of ripping apart meat with greasy bare hands and feeding morsels to one's partner as well as being fed oneself does have its effects. On the other hand, if you believe that the powdered horn of a white rhinoceros can help you, then the belief may do so,.. not the rhinoceros horn.

Altogether weird and wonderful things have often been tried. Cartolomeo Scappi was cook to Pope Pius V. Why he should need to invent an aphrodisiac for a religious figure sworn to the extreme perversion of celibacy is unknown to me, but his recipe depended on the testicles of bulls. No less an authority than Pliny the Elder and also Horace mention the use of marinated sow vulvas as powerfully effective. One cannot but remark that no wonder the Romans conquered the known world if their determination in battle equalled their courageous singleness of purpose in the devouring of sow's vulvas.

Unfortunate though it is, we must conclude that none of these odd ideas work. Alcohol in small quantities helps a little, perhaps by lowering the inhibitions. Marijuana seems to do the same but with less danger. The use of cocaine as a sexual stimulant has recently become popular, but it is expensive, illegal, and over indulgence can be harmful. The secrets of the real things,.. satyrion, stramonium, bufotenine and such, must be sought in other books as already mentioned above. They are easy and cheap to find, simple to use, and perfectly safe under appropriate conditions. Sadly enough the facts are that apart from the things mentioned above, as the cynic once said, 'The only real aphrodisiac in the world is money',... though some contend that it is power.

Footnote: In recent years a homoeopathic product has been developed in Switzerland which many report to have sexually stimulating effects. It was originally intended as an overall enhancement to the sexual system in general and has proved very effective indeed as such. The manufacturers regard any aphrodisiac effects as mere bonus. Called Masculone (there is also Feminone for women) it is referred to in greater detail in a later section.

\* \* \*

## Chapter Eight: Penis Rituals and Phallic Worship

### The tribal penis

During man's first faltering steps towards civilisation he subsisted by being a hunter-gatherer. Men hunted for food from animal sources whenever available. The club, the spear and later the arrow were the hunting tools. The similarity of those tools with a penis was apparent even to the simplest mind. The women and children, and during hard times, the men too supplemented provisions by gathering fruit, seeds and roots, and edible material from the animal world like eggs, and honey whenever they could. Here too men were strong and dominant. Women were their inferiors at least on this level. The importance and authority of the penis bearer was absolute.

Other experts have seen the sequence differently. They take as their starting point not the primitive hunting peoples but, later on, the first dawn of agriculture when man sought to make his supplies more certain by growing them instead of relying on the choice between lucky finds and empty bellies. The early work in agriculture was largely done by women. The tasks were light but menial, hoeing, clearing weeds and so on. Much as in today's suburban garden many tasks were beneath the power and dignity of men. So women were in a sense important contributors. They too actually brought forth the new humans from within themselves in the awe-inspiring, dangerous and frightening process of childbirth. Particularly in the Middle East this joint association of childbirth and food-providing made women the prominent figures in fertility rites at least for a time. The next step changed all that; man actually started breaking open the ground to prepare it for planting. The plough was invented. That needed strength to hold it below the ground and, in the absence of beasts of burden, to haul it through the earth. The plough's symbolic association of strength, breaking open and preparing for seed was also a parallel with the penis too obvious to be missed. The male organ quickly assumed its position of dominance.

### The mystical penis

The actual sequence of events is not only uncertain but is, apart from academically, unimportant. By whatever means, the penis became a natural object of adoration and religious fervour. The phenomenon of Phallic Worship had arrived. Neither was it restricted to the Middle East. Throughout the ancient world it spread or made its spontaneous appearance. Not only the eastern world was involved. With the spread of peoples it also crossed the ice-bound Bering Straits with the forerunners of the North American Indians perhaps twenty or thirty thousand years ago. The phallic pillars of the Yucatan were there long before white people came. So were the phallic heads of Easter Island. The worship of the sexual organs as generative in their ability and a repository of creative power became world-wide. It can be seen from the eastern worship of Lingam-Yoni to the great god Baal of Canaan, from Japan to Ephesus and even to the carved symbol of an erect penis in a church in Bordeaux, France. Phallic worship has ebbed and flowed as a religious source, but even to this very day in London is a group that meets regularly for its own particular rites of penis worship. Many of the rites are flagrantly sexual in their execution and the group is in contact with other groups elsewhere both within the country and abroad.

One of the oldest symbols of the penis according to some authorities is the Ankh. Mostly this is found on the relief carvings of the Egyptian tombs and temples. Widely regarded as a symbolic penis and by others as a symbol of life, the distinction between the two is small. It is commonly seen in the hands of pharaohs or gods and in particular being held to the lips of the people represented. The connection between this symbolic act and the fertility effects of the penis inserted into the mouth and especially ejaculating there (See Chapter Five) will not be overlooked. The Ankh, also known as the Crux-Ansata, is not restricted to Egypt. It exists in even earlier carvings in Ninevah and later on in Indian cave temples. The strong influence of phallicism in the Hindu mind is well recognised today. Another symbol of the penis worshippers is the present Maltese Cross. Nowadays this is shown by four identical triangles, joined at their apices to form a cross each with a notch in the side away from the cross. Previously the sign was made up of four erect penises touching at the glans and was changed only when the symbol was adopted as a religious symbol centuries later. The change from the testicles' twin-bulges to the notched triangle is very clear when the two symbols are seen together. Amongst others, the familiar black and white uniformed First Aid teams of St. John's Ambulance Brigade wear this symbol today. It seems unlikely that they are familiar with its origin!

### The worshipped penis

Phallic worship is an exceedingly old religious process. No one knows where or how it started; almost certainly it was not always the spread of an idea, but the spontaneous occurrence of the same idea in different places. Some things are so universal and, to the primitive mind, so obviously a likely subject for worship that they occur independently to scattered peoples. Worship of the sun is perhaps the most natural of all. It seems possible that penis worship preceded even this or was at least contemporary with it. Irrespective of arguments about dating, one thing is very sure. In early, comparatively uncivilised communities there was no association between the penis, sexual rites, and so on and any aspect of immorality. Indeed, the reverse was true. Penis worship was aimed at and was part of the vital expansion of population. As such it and all fertility processes were highly desirable. To a large extent it was with the rise of Judaism and Christianity that sex developed its 'dirty' associations and began to be deliberately exploited and therefore misunderstood.

### The Biblical Penis

The worship of sex and the penis was partly its fertility connection. No doubt too it was partly because of the intense pleasure of sexual contact, which no other human phenomenon can anywhere near approach, that the worship of both male and female genitalia arose. No one thought of it as evil, dirty or undesirable. Even the Hebrew God, and other gods before him, decreed that men and women should be fruitful and multiply. It follows from this dictum that this stern and jealous god, who openly demonstrated a number of the least pleasant characteristics of mankind, not only did not criticise but looked with favour upon sexual indulgence. Indeed, it seems that it was one of the few really nice things that gods always approved of. It is true that things like homosexuality and bestiality were heavily punishable. After all, these sexual practices were not productive; there was no resultant fertility. But things went much further than that. Not only was fertility positively encouraged but lack of fertility was deprecated. In the Book of Deuteronomy (Ch.23 v.1) we find that if a man, through no fault of his own, was "wounded in the stones" that is the testicles, or if he was unfortunate enough to suffer loss of the penis, say in battle, then from that day he was to be ostracised. From then on he could no longer be allowed even to "enter into the congregation of the Lord." And in

Genesis 38 v.9 we read that Onan was actually slain for what some have thought to be masturbation but was more likely to have been coitus interruptus.

Comments concerning the importance of the phallus and phallic objects abound in the Bible. Jacob, for example, (Genesis 28), built a pillar of stones as an act of worship. On the top of this phallic symbol he then poured oil (semen). In Psalm 92 we read that "... the Lord is upright and is a rock." Small wonder that the Hebrews, like Neolithic people in Salisbury Plain, should raise upright rocks as emblems of the power of the penis. For the Hebrews, however, the symbol was only of or for the God. It was never the God himself. Retribution awaited those who carried the identification too far, whatever their station in life. In 1 Kings 15 (and 2 Chronicles, 14) we read that King Asa dethroned his queen mother for presiding in sacrifices to some priapic deity.

**The fertile penis**

Elsewhere these subtle niceties were not important. In Dahomey hollow models of the god Legba are made with the penis rigid and prominent. This is filled with palm oil which is allowed to drip slowly out through the penis tip. Would-be mothers pray to the god as a fertility rite. The god's semen, the sacred palm oil, becomes significant too in sacred cooking, body cleansing and to make balms to rub into the male and female genitalia before and during sexual activities.

In some old temples dedicated to phallic gods, the carved wooden god was so frequently visited by barren and hopeful women that the wood of the penis wore down from the handling, kissing, sucking and rubbing to which it was repeatedly subjected. The temple priests solved the problem by making the phallus out of the tip of the shaft of a long piece of wood protruding through a hole between the God's thighs. As the penis wore away they simply went behind the statue when all was quiet and hammered the shaft a few inches further through from behind.

It was the practice of the Romans to celebrate the arrival of spring with fertility rites. During these, large models of a penis were carried around the fields that were soon to be ploughed. This finds a parallel in the ancient English custom of 'beating the bounds.' In this, groups of men walk around the limits of the parish striking its borders with wooden sticks, telling lewd jests, singing rude songs and carrying logs and loaves baked into cylinders. The reasons behind these phallic- and cylindrically-shaped images have been largely forgotten but their origins were real enough in their day. In parts of Spain even nowadays the coming of spring is celebrated at midnight on St. Joseph's Day by the festival of the Fallus or Fallas. Spellings, derivations and associations of both the word and the event vary but huge bonfires in the streets consume statues that have been on display and many of which are flagrantly sexual in style.

For the Romans things were much more extreme. During their spring fertility feastings, their activities were characterised by every species of lewd debauchery suggested by the inflamed imaginations of the riotous and drunken adherents. Normally quiet and gentle women, desperate in their thwarted attempts to become pregnant, copulated repeatedly in the streets with total strangers and without the restraint of their menfolk. Others threw themselves in frenzy at the phallic gods, hung garlands of flowers on them and sat astride those with exaggerated, tree trunk-like penises, rubbing and tearing at them until their genitals were sore and bleeding. Maidens too climbed onto other gods of more realistic proportions. There they squatted and copulated with the god so that it should be first to dispose of their modesty and in order that they should thus become fertile and treasured by their future husbands.

The ancient customs of fertilising the spring ploughing and grazing fields with semen still exists. Usually at the first full moon after the winter solstice the village men masturbate into a freshly turned spadeful of soil or a freshly ploughed furrow. Sometimes this ritual is varied by the local women who are voluntarily subjected to intercourse while hands and feet are buried in, or clutching at the soil. Then, as part of the same ritual a black cock and a white hen, tied together like a man and a woman copulating, have their throats cut simultaneously. Their mingled blood is scattered on the ground and their still-tied bodies are then buried traditionally at the highest point of the land. To this writer's certain knowledge these rituals have been performed in Kent, Dorset and Gwent within the last decade!

**The Satanic Penis**

The connection of magic with fertility is not restricted to agriculture. Sexual contact between humans and animals is also recorded, the intention being similar. Satanic rites, most of which have sexual features, are commonly corrupted fertility rituals. In them, humans often copulate with animals or animal effigies. In particular women submit to trained dogs in acts of submission or to a goat representing Satan himself. Whether it is an animal or the Dark Priest himself who actually copulates, his enthusiasm and capacity for sustained intercourse with so many women quickly wanes. Thereupon a symbolic thrusting device,.. usually a stone dildo, is pressed into multiple service. In spite of the frenzy of the orgies that are associated with satanic, magical rites, this probably explains why participants usually describe the sexual response of the Devil as being cold and his organ as being chilly and unyielding.

It should not be thought that these ancient spells and rituals all belong in the past. Satanic and other mystical covens abound nowadays in most civilised countries. The activities of many of them are beyond obscene and, again to this writer's certain knowledge, are so infamous as to constitute criminally punishable offences as they are well outside what the law would permit even for religious purposes.

The connection between some traditions of fertility symbolism, even in the modern British population is often not recognised but it is as present as it ever was. The reasons are lost, or at any rate unrealised, by the people who carry them out. There are nonetheless plenty of fertility phenomena to be observed in most households. Examples are baking pastry (or gingerbread) people, turning one's money over when the moon is new, bringing catkins into the house in spring and fir trees and red berries in winter, kissing beneath the mistletoe, cutting the hair when the moon is waning, and many, many others. You can find plenty of examples if you look. Throwing the bride's posy to the bridesmaids, scattering confetti, (symbolic grain) and placing a symbolic vulva on the bride's fourth finger are just some that are connected with marriage. And on the village green in the long, warm evenings young girls and sometimes men too, dance with ribbons around the phallic shaft of the Maypole, an object found in similar form in the South Sea Islands, the British Columbian forests and the Deccan of India.

Not all such activities surrounding the all-important sexual organs of men and women are of such harmless and attractive characteristics as the majority of these fertility rites. A darker side shows itself in the way men and less often women have treated the genitalia in such a way as to restrict their use. In some unexplained way human jealousies are greatest of all when involved with sex. A man is jealous of his woman. He is disturbed if another man looks at her. He is worried if she looks at another man. He is furious if there is some clandestine contact between them. He may be suicidal or homicidal if that contact is an actively genital one. In some exaggerated way the genitals are more important than love, affection, devotion and all the other parts of the body together.

In this day and age such behaviour patterns are quite irrational. They exist just the same, and it is as well for the most balanced mind to recognise that it can be shaken or even demolished by these immense forces should they ever be released.

**Secret sexual rites**

In an attempt to prevent such a likelihood, various techniques have been resorted to in other times and places. The women of some tribes perforate the man's foreskin and, if he is to be away from the village for a while, sew it loosely together with leather thongs. The thongs are closed with a secret knot known only to the old women of the group. Under these circumstances erection is too painful to contemplate and even nocturnal emission is rare. This preserves not only the valuable semen but the privately owned quality of the penis until the return of the man from his hunting or fighting sortie.

This protection is more often encountered for the preservation of the female 'honour.' Chastity belts, some of which are of fearsome ingenuity and some of which are worn mostly symbolically and for fun even today, could always be opened by a sufficiently persistent application of ingenuity. Not so the vulva of the infibulated woman. For this a number of methods were available. The labia might be pierced by permanent holes which could be closed by secret knots and seals if the couple were to be parted. Alternatively, a vaginal plug could be inserted and fastened securely in position to make the space unavailable. Most brutal of all was the technique of lacerating the labia of an infant girl then sewing them together so that they healed closed with only a tiny aperture for urination. When the first menstrual blood appeared the girl, always a guaranteed virgin, would be betrothed at a savage initiation ceremony. The vulva was laid open by the excruciatingly painful severing apart of the labia by a ceremonial knife.

Sometimes an even more vicious motive lay behind the mutilation. A way was sought to make a women less sexually arousable. The technique is often mistakenly called female circumcision. Circumcision of the female is possible. It involves cutting away part of the female foreskin, the tiny cloak of skin covering the clitoris. Usually, however, what is meant by female circumcision is actually the removal of the entire clitoris and its foreskin and often a substantial portion of the inner labia too. This is more correctly called clitoridectomy. The girl, often drugged and pinioned, has the area grasped and slashed off by a series of cuts with a knife, old razor blade or even a sharp fragment of shattered glass. The area is then bound up to heal. This method, still used in north east Africa, can cause loss of life by haemorrhage and infection. To avoid this, another way is to tie the girl, widely splayed, then apply the glowing end of a hot ember directly to the clitoris. Amid great pain it disappears forever and with it its alleged problems.

The entire question of circumcision, male and female, raises a number of highly significant problems. Why, after all, should such an action be invented at all? And of all places, why the genitals? Max Gluckman in his *Essays on the Ritual of Social Relations* mentions clitoridectomy as removing that part of the female that resembles the male. Conversely male circumcision removes that part which could be held vaguely to look similar to that vulva. It is certainly true that some women, when asked to explain their preferences for circumcised or uncircumcised men, will say that they regard the uncircumcised penis as feminine-looking and they like or dislike it accordingly. I have also heard men say that the absence of their foreskin makes them feel in some way diminished,.. as if the missing foreskin makes them look smaller. It is true in my experience that more circumcised men ask about the possibilities of undergoing penis enlargement than do uncircumcised men.

Whatever the originating and underlying causes, it is undoubtedly true that circumcision has a lot more to it than the equivalent idea of chopping half an inch of the exhaust-pipe of a new car. Some influential black African leaders have advised white action groups and doctors not to interfere by trying to eliminate (particularly female) circumcision. They contend that it is a deep-rooted and significant social phenomena amongst the tribes that do it and something vital to the identification of the individual as a group member, and so on. It could be similarly argued that vital cohesive social forces now surround the practice of male circumcision in the Jewish community. Yet so familiar is it that few would attempt to curtail that practice. Whatever the original reasons claimed for circumcision, male or female, socio-religious forces do now surround them the obstruction of which could have unpredictable results. Caution is clearly needed rather than outright and unguided attack.

It may have been the fundamental importance of the penis as a body part that led to its being chosen as the site of the visible extraction of the Blood of the Covenant that formed, as it were, the contract between the Hebrews and their nomadic god. Nowadays it remains as essential as ever. Only twice in a professional lifetime have I known a Jewish man to enquire about plastic surgery to refashion his missing prepuce.

**Jewish law and the penis**

The technique of Jewish ritual circumcision is very well documented by Jacob Snowman MD, MRCP, in a book first written in 1904 but repeatedly republished since. Generally the act is carried out by a Mohel who must himself be an adult, circumcised Jew, and an adherent of Judaism. Within the religion it is obligatory for every Jewish father to ensure that his son is circumcised. If the father doesn't or is unavailable, the duty falls on the religious authorities. If all else fails the duty falls to the child himself, at the age of thirteen, to present himself for circumcision.

The operation, which is customarily carried out on the eighth day of life and before sunset, is in a number of stages. First the area is very thoroughly cleaned. Such washing commonly causes erection. If not, erection can be induced. (This act of erection in the new-born is also commonly done in Christian communities often by the midwife. Alternatively the mother or a female relative may do it by hand, or commonly by sucking). A special shield with a hole is slipped over the penis so that the slack of the foreskin can be drawn through while the glans is held safely back out of the way. The foreskin is then sliced away. The mucous membrane lining the foreskin is torn back to free it. Now takes place perhaps the most vital part of the ritual, the Metzizah. Formerly this was done by taking the penis in the mouth and sucking it. Nowadays in the interest of hygiene a glass tube, some three inches long and three quarters of an inch in diameter, is used. It is placed over the penis, pushed tight to seal it against the abdominal wall, and the open end is then sucked. The important thing is that the penis must bleed. It is this act which accomplishes the drawing of the blood of the Covenant. Without it the circumcision is not valid. The mucous membrane and severed foreskin remnants are then so positioned that they can heal properly and the area is adequately dressed. So significant is this ritual that it must never be omitted. True, if a mother or father has lost two sons from the effects of circumcision they must wait until the third one is older before risking it. However, should a babe die before it is circumcised then its corpse should still have its foreskin amputated before burial.

As mentioned above, there is much discussion concerning the pros and cons of circumcision in the modern world. I make no comment on the deed as a religious ritual as I do not have a religion and am in no way qualified to criticise. There are some medical/surgical reasons why circumcision may be required, e.g. a very tight foreskin. Such reasons are, however, fairly uncommon and only something up to five per cent of males are likely to need it. The others should be left alone if only on the grounds that if something is OK. you don't fool with it. ['If it ain't broke don't fix it!'] Perhaps, as some argue, the over-exposed glans is rendered less sensitive. That may be bad in one way, but it may enable a man to prolong intercourse. Perhaps the absence of the foreskin keeps the glans cleaner by rubbing the smegma off onto the clothing. On the other hand soap and water clean it just as well and without the risk of picking up germs from the clothing. Smegma can cause cancer of the female uterus (in a most minute number of cases). Once again soap and water remove it. Some women do derive a kind of deep matriarchal satisfaction from leaving a permanently irremovable mark on the sexual organ of their offspring.

Some men and women will describe their preference for the 'Roundhead' or the 'Cavalier' by saying, "I know what I like." In reality this is rather like the way they answer a similar question about music. The answer really means, "I like what I know," so it is just about as reliable. My own feeling is that as the operation is reversible only partially, with difficulty and by expensive plastic surgery, it is far better not to circumcise in infancy. A man can always decide for himself later. It is one of the sober duties of a parent to keep as many options open to the offspring as possible. The option to have or not have a foreskin should most certainly be included in these.

All in all it would appear an anachronism nowadays to regard as vital the barbaric process of insisting that a helpless baby should have its sexual organ injured until it bleeds in order to achieve a religious status. If it is to be condoned, there would appear to be no logical reason for not also condoning female circumcision. (This is an illegal operation in UK and many other countries). One cannot but wonder whether, had it been the removal of an eyelid or two that the deity fancied, the idea,.. and even that particularly demanding deity, might never have caught on?

**Adorning the penis**

The modern man is not altogether without some ways of adorning his penis. Some of these are mentioned in greater length in Chapter Fifteen. Here though, in the discussion on penis surgery techniques, must be mentioned the current fashion for Erotic Piercing or Body Piercing as it sometimes termed. Nowadays there is an increasing tendency for men to wear decorations in the penis and nipples and for women to wear their similar decorations in nipples, navel and labia.

The foreskin is very suitable for piercing and a variety of rings or studs can be inserted. Such rings can also be worn through the nipples though more often men choose barbells for this purpose. Very popular too is the famous Prince Albert Ring, so named as one was allegedly worn, to considerable effect it is said, by no less a person than the Prince Consort of Queen Victoria! Correctly positioned this ring runs through the floor of the urethra up to two centimetres inside the meatus, from which orifice it then emerges. It gives a fascinating and aggressively masculine look especially to the erect organ and, it is claimed, adds immensely to both male and female sensation during the in-and-out frictions of intercourse.

Women more often choose rings rather than barbells for their nipples as they are more suitable for attaching light chains and such, worn during fetishistic and mildly sado-masochistic sex games. Simple rings or earrings through the labia or even the clitoris itself are also becoming more and more popular. [Note: legislation against female circumcision is, in some areas, widely interpreted also to include any form of mutilation of the clitoris and labia. Erotic piercing may be held to infringe such rigid application. Those carrying out the procedure should therefore be aware of this risk as the consent of the 'patient' does not, of itself, constitute any right to break the law].

Regrettably there are a number of quack operators performing these piercings and these are mentioned only in order to be roundly condemned. Erotic piercing is very safe and very easy but only if done by a properly trained and qualified physician of experience. The doctor will know the anatomy, avoid accidental severing of blood vessels, use correct instruments and techniques and work with full aseptic procedure. (A confidential and discreet clinic that carries out such procedures is mentioned in the Sources List). A pin-prick for the local anaesthetic is the only momentary instant of pain the patient will detect. After that the piercing can be carried out slowly and meticulously and with no further discomfort. The entire procedure is over in minutes and proper instructions on aftercare given.

All kinds and varieties of decorations are now in use. Some people have a considerable number of rings that can be removed as easily as earrings. Occasionally, with couples, two rings are inserted in the foreskin of the man and one in each of his partner's labia. These pairs are then closed by a tiny padlock and the keys exchanged as tokens of the ensured fidelity. The variety of piercings and the games played with them is simply enormous.

* * *

# SECTION THREE:
# THE BROKEN PENIS

**Chapter Nine:** Diseases of the Penis

The penis can become diseased, damaged or dysfunctional by either psychological or physical means or both. The psychological problems are, generally speaking, the sexual problems that beset human relationships. They and their solutions will be dealt with in depth in the two subsequent chapters. Physical causes are disease processes. As such they fall naturally into two groups; generalised diseases, or those situated other than in the genital organs but affecting them just the same, and diseases specifically of or taking place in the sexual equipment itself.

**Prime causes of penis malfunction**

Some of the conditions classed as generalised diseases are indeed not so much diseases as self-induced habits. Foremost amongst these is obesity. Obesity lowers the libido and sexual ability. The fat person, in addition to having actual technical difficulty with intercourse from the physical presence of extra fat layers getting in the way of positions and flexibility, can find that exercise capacity is reduced by the tiredness and breathlessness resulting from exertion. Alcoholism is another problem. Whereas a drink or two may sharpen the appetite, lift the spirits and enhance the libido, a larger quantity does the opposite. It has long been known that although alcohol increases the desires, it decreases the performance. This is especially true of the repeated consumer of large amounts. Going home from a party with pulse racing and loins itching for action from the effect of alcohol all too often ends up with a total inability to raise an erection when the bed is reached. [Joke: a cocktail party is an occasion where the men stand around getting stiff and the women stand around getting tight, and when they get home neither is either!]

Diabetes is another condition in which sexual capacity is commonly, thought not always impaired. Some drugs too can have a depressing effect. The tricyclics so widely used in the therapy of emotional disorders are big offenders. So are some of the drugs used to reduce blood pressure. All too many doctors automatically assume that dangerous conditions like blood pressure should have priority over sexual inclinations. This is not always the patient's preferred option. Doctors should always have regard to the patient's priorities and should elicit them before a mutual decision with regard to therapy is arrived at. There are usually alternatives to the chosen drugs if these prove to have sexual side-effects. If you are concerned about the effects on your sex life, it would be as well to discuss their use in detail with your medical adviser before embarking on a long course of treatment.

The importance of heart disease is something that produces plenty of questions from patients. The rule of thumb is that if the extent of the heart disease is such that it permits the patient to walk half a mile or climb two flights of stairs it will permit the non-strenuous type of intercourse. Even within a few weeks of a coronary attack, the degree of progress should be such that gentle masturbation or oral sex should be not only safe but positively beneficial to the morale of the patient. Clearly, very strenuous activities of all types are unsuitable and this includes sex. The redevelopment of sexual performance should be a part of the overall general return to activity after the acute phases of heart disease recede.

Disease of the sex organs important enough to require a mention here are so many that we shall deal with them in alphabetical order.

**Balanitis:** This is the inflammation of the glans. It can be an exceedingly painful condition. Because of this it seldom escapes medical attention and therefore proper treatment. Probably the chief cause is bad hygiene. Smegma collecting, unwashed, inside the foreskin harbours bacteria which set up infection. Washing every day with ordinary soap and water is the safeguard.

**Diphallus:** A very rare condition but worth mentioning for its novelty. It is the congenital condition of the man with two penises. They are invariably side by side. Most such anomalies exist only with such severe accompanying faults in the rest of the urogenital system as to be incompatible with life.

**'Fracture' of the penis:** This is not a true fracture in the accepted sense of the word as no bone is involved, there being no bones in the penis. The penis at its maximum degree of erection is extremely rigid. It is attached firmly at the root and for several inches in front of that, to both bones and sheets of ligament and muscle. If during erection it is forcibly wrenched or twisted, especially in a downward direction, so-called fracture may result. Such actions may be the result of over-zealous activity by the female partner. More often the cause is being in an unstable position of intercourse when one of other partner slips, thereby pulling fiercely on the shaft. The actual injury is a rupture of a corpus cavernosum (see Chapter 1). Blood, under pressure, oozes out from the wound into other tissues of the penis and the perineum. There is usually considerable pain. The only treatment for this is surgical so get to the nearest casualty department. Don't delay. An ice-cold compress helps a little in the meantime.

**Granuloma:** This is not the same as lymphogranuloma (see below) but may look similar. A tender, red, hardish patch appears somewhere on or near the genitalia. It forms a sore which becomes swollen, discharging and ulcer-like. Like all such unexplained conditions, you should seek medical advice. [Joke: there really was once a breakfast cereal given this name. It did not catch on!].

**Growths:** These are of two kinds, malignant and non-malignant. Malignant ones are not common and there is no way to describe them properly here. The benign ones are called papillomata, or love warts. They are like single or clustered groups of tiny warts or skin tags usually on the shaft of the penis just behind the coronal groove. They can spread, including from one person to another during sexual contact, and are probably caused by a virus. The treatment is simple with Podophyllin or other application but is better used under medical supervision.

**Herpes:** This is also a virus infection and usually appears on the glans or the foreskin. It starts off resembling the typical herpes, like a cold sore near the mouth, with a cluster of small watery blisters. These soon burst and leave a tender, red area of erosion. As long as it doesn't get a secondary infection it is self-healing in 7-10 days. Unfortunately the infection then seldom disappears but merely lies dormant. Over a period of many years it can reappear, particularly in response to sexual activity. It may appear once a month or once a year. It is nearly always painful and is very highly infectious. As a result of this and as, at this stage, it is virtually incurable, it is often enough to put an end to a person's sex life once and for all. The social implications of catching an unconcealable herpes are obvious enough.

**Hydrocoele:** This is the condition in which the scrotum becomes swollen as it fills up with a watery fluid. It is not dangerous but the scrotum can become so huge that the penis is literally lost in it. It almost never gets better on its own and treatment depends either on having it drained at the required intervals (a technique you can be taught to do yourself) or upon having it operated on and cured permanently. The snag with a hydrocoele, apart from the inconvenience of its size and unseemly appearance, is that inside it there may also be a hernia. This could remain undetected for a long time and is a possible danger that should not be neglected.

**Hypospadias:** A congenital condition which is surprisingly common, perhaps affecting one man in 350. The orifice (meatus) of the urethra, instead of being more or less at or just above the centre of the glans tip is situated below it. It may be only a little displaced from the normal position but can be well down underneath where the frenum of the foreskin is attached and with the glans bulging over the top. For the most part it is not a serious sexual handicap, erection and intercourse being scarcely different from the usual. Some distortions however can be severe and a source of embarrassment, particularly where the meatus is somewhere under the shaft of the penis or even further down on the perineum and urination and ejaculation therefore take place from there. The further back the orifice, the more the tendency of the penis shaft to have a pronounced downward curve (called 'bowing'). The entire condition can be the cause of sexual and social problems. It can usually be most elegantly repaired by good plastic surgery and advice about this should preferably be taken early in infancy.

**Infection:** Smegma coming from the tiny glands around the foreskin has, mixed with it, dead cells cast off from the skin. As the penis is frequently handled, and anyway hangs outside the body, bacteria continuously collect in the smegma. Disease-causing bacteria have thus an ideal chance of growing and setting up an infection. The thing that helps this undesirable process most is stagnation, or in other words, allowing the infected smegma to go on collecting and lying undisturbed inside the foreskin. It is only a question of time before that causes trouble. The answer is hygiene. The circumcised male has no problem, but the uncircumcised should draw the foreskin back and rinse away the stale smegma with soap and water at least once daily. One word of warning. The aroma of smegma is erotic to a lot of women. So just before intercourse is most surely the wrong time to wash it if your partner is one of these. An hour or so before is far better.

**Lymphogranuloma:** This is really a virus disease of tropical climates and is venereal; that is, it spreads by sexual contact. It used to be rarely seen in Europe or America but with contemporary wide movements of population it is becoming more common. It starts off looking a bit like a cold sore on the genitals. It is short lasting and not painful. A month later one or more glands swell in one or both groins. These may grow up to a couple of inches long, burst through the skin, and form a discharging sinus. Treatment is not difficult but it is useless to put creams or ointments on it yourself. It needs the VD clinic.

**Meatal stenosis:** This may be congenital or acquired. It is the narrowing of the urethral opening at the glans tip. Congenital cases are usually spotted early by the parents. It can also follow such operations as circumcision. If the hole is very narrow (called a pin-hole meatus) there can result a back pressure on the rest of the urinary system. This causes damage. The condition needs a simple operation to correct it.

**Orchitis:** Inflammation of the testicles. Every man knows how tender a testicle is if struck or squeezed too hard. Apart from the few disturbed masochists for whom hurting the testicles is a sexual turn-on, no one likes testicular pain. Inflammation with its associated swelling is very painful indeed. It can come as a result of prolonged erection or lying awkwardly, perhaps in tight clothing. The tubes that drain the normal body fluids [lymph] away from the testicles are compressed and don't allow proper drainage. The testicles swell slightly and become very painful. This is the condition known as 'lover's nuts' or as 'blue balls.' The only solution (apart from prevention) is to go to bed with a couple of aspirins and, if possible, a light suspensory bandage to support the scrotum. By morning the swelling and pain should have disappeared. This mechanical orchitis is temporary and without after effects. A more important and prolonged orchitis may result from serious injury or secondary to infection elsewhere as, for example, in mumps. A long spell of pain and extreme tenderness may leave permanent damage to the testicles and result in sterility. As the chances of complications are worse later in life, it is as well to make sure your son gets mumps in the comparative safety of infancy.

**Phimosis and paraphimosis:** The former is the inflammation of the foreskin, usually from under-lying smegma-born infection and when the foreskin opening is very narrow. If the tight foreskin is drawn right back behind the glans it may cause the glans to swell so that the foreskin forms a tight band around the penis in the region of the coronal groove. If this state of affairs persists for long (an hour or so) it becomes impossible to pull the foreskin forward over the glans again. The resulting inflammation and swelling is paraphimosis. Sometimes a painful paraphimosis can be relieved by the doctor's technique of compressing the swollen glans until it slips back within the foreskin. This is a temporary measure. Whereas repeated working and stretching of the foreskin may be sufficient to loosen it adequately (especially in an infant), in the adult it is more likely that the correct treatment is full circumcision. In acute cases of paraphimosis, circumcision may have to be an emergency procedure. Never delay with this condition. Get help before permanent serious damage results from the restricted blood supply.

**Peyronie's disease:** This is a fairly uncommon but seriously handicapping disease of the penis. The cause is largely unknown. Usually starting after the age of 40 the first thing noticed is a tendency of the penis to curve more during erection. Erection also starts to become painful. On feeling the soft organ it is often possible to detect one or more hard patches on the upper surface of one or other corpus cavernosum. The condition is usually progressive, and over a period of years the penis may become grossly distorted with a number of lumps, bumps and twists in it. It may become sexually unusable. Worst of all is when the pain becomes an important factor, though as a rule this tends to decrease rather than increase. At present treatment is far from always successful but medical help is certainly indicated.

**Priapism:** Opinions vary as to whether this is ever a psychological problem or always a pathological one. The condition of persistent, painful and unwanted erection (not the same as the pleasant one that arrives in dreams or on waking), is usually due to the veins that drain blood away from the penis becoming blocked generally near the prostate gland. Relief usually depends on surgery.

**Prostate gland problems:** As a man gets older so his prostate gland tends to enlarge. It is seldom that this is not the case, though very often the degree of enlargement is not enough to cause serious trouble. The condition is called benign prostatic hypertrophy

[BPH] and, more than anything else, its problems are mechanical. The usual difficulty is that, being situated around the first part of the urethra, enlargement of the prostate can impede the passage of urine. It may well need surgery, either being shaved down a bit or radically removed. The fear is that the latter operation (called prostatectomy) may cause a subsequent and permanent lack of erection. This can happen, especially if the surgeon permits extensive damage to the blood vessels in the area. Different surgeons have different techniques and the results of some are better than others in this field. For example, the Madigan type of operation is usually better from this aspect than the more common Millen operation. Correctly done, prostatectomy need not affect erection other than temporarily. So, if it matters to you, shop around for your surgeon and make a point of telling him, preferably in writing, of what you do and do not consent to. After all he only wants your prostate. Why should he have your erection too?

Cancer of the prostate gland has become more common in recent years, probably as the population has aged. It is now a substantial cause of cancer deaths. Sometimes there is preceding inflammation,.. prostatitis, with some discomfort, some sexual difficulty like uncomfortable ejaculation and the passage of small amounts of blood in the semen. The success rates of treatment by surgery or by chemotherapy and/or radiotherapy are quite good especially if the condition is detected early and treated by an expert. Whatever symptoms are experienced in this zone they merit early attention by skilled medical practitioners.

**Stones:** These are not common but do occur particularly in later life. Perhaps an old man loses his partner and his sex interest. He ceases, perhaps for some years, ever to draw back the foreskin. The smegma, if it does not become infected, can become hard and formed into near solid chunk. The stone can rub and cause pain and ulcers. Proper manipulation of the foreskin and adequate washing is the prevention and these precautions should never be neglected, irrespective of sexual requirement, from the cradle to the grave.

**Undescended testicle:** During the time that the baby boy spends growing inside the mother's uterus, his testicles develop well inside his own body. Gradually, as birth approaches, they move out from his abdomen through overlapping holes in the muscles of his abdominal wall near the groins. Suspended by a thick chord of muscle containing the blood vessels, nerves and the vas, etc. each testicle descends into the scrotum. It normally reaches this position shortly before birth. Should it not do so, but get held up part way, it is called an undescended testicle. (If it descends but in the wrong direction, it is a maldescended testicle). Most baby boys are routinely examined to check for this condition. If one testicle is undescended to start with it will often descend of its own accord a little later. If not, some hormone treatment may help it on its way or if all else fails it can be put into the scrotum surgically. One thing is worth mentioning. Even if you have only one testicle, it is more than enough to ensure all the adequate production of sperms and sex hormones. Indeed, in men who lose one testicle the other may well increase in size to help compensate. Losing one ball doesn't mean you should lose heart. It won't curb your manhood.

**Urethritis:** Inflammation of the urethra. The inside of the tube becomes tender and gives off a thin liquid discharge. This can be squeezed out to appear at the meatus especially if no urine has been passed for some time. An example of this is first thing in the morning when the discharge so observed is known as 'the morning drop.' Sometimes the cause is one particular infectious organism (bacteria) as in gonorrhoea (see below). At other times it can be more of a group of germs and the condition is then spoken of as N.S.U. or non-specific urethritis. Sometimes it is caught by picking up the infected germ from a vagina (or mouth, or hand) that already has it. Other times it is more of a mechanical nature from the repeated friction that goes with long sexual sessions or intercourse at very frequent intervals. Together with the discharge there is a sensation of a hot, piercing pain up through the shaft of the penis. This is particularly painful during the passing of urine and can be so excruciating that it is likened to passing 'powdered glass, razor blades and old car tyres.' Infection may spread back into the bladder thus causing cystitis and giving rise to the added symptoms of urgency (the need to urinate very quickly) and frequency (an increase in the number of times urine needs to be passed), and worst of all strangury (a frantic and overwhelming desire to pass urine which nonetheless only passes with difficulty or in exceedingly painful dribbles). NSU is easily treated and cured, but there is a need to distinguish it from real gonorrhoea. Treatment at a VD centre is therefore always recommended.

**Varicocoele:** This might be described as having varicose veins not on the legs but in the walls of the scrotum. The veins are distended and give the surface a blue marked and gnarled surface. There is little danger but it is unsightly and can cause a prolonged discomfort known as 'drag' from its sheer weight. Surgical treatment is easy and comparatively painless.

**Venereal diseases [VD]:** In theory this is any kind of disease spread by any kind of sexual contact. In practice, however, apart from the more unusual things like lymphogranuloma (above) and more recently the AIDS epidemic, it really means two conditions, syphilis and gonorrhoea.

Syphilis is far less common but far more serious. It has increased in recent years, probably because of the arrival of the Permissive Society. It is interesting to note however that gonorrhoea has increased far more in the same time. This raises the question as to whether or not other relevant influential factors may be at work as well as merely the alleged promiscuity. Only very few syphilis germs (called treponema) need to infect an area to set up the start of the disease. Infection is usually via the genitals simply because they are most used for sexual contact. With the increase in oral sex the mouth is also nowadays more frequently seen to be infected. Amongst homosexuals particularly the anal region can be involved. Spread of the disease is very fast. Although the early effects are virtually harmless and almost unnoticed, the later effects are utterly destructive over a large area of the body. Inadequately treated, it seriously incapacitates one victim in five and kills one in ten. The first sign, between two and six weeks after infection, is a little painless spot at the original point of entry. This is called a primary chancre and there are usually some swollen glands nearby. At about six weeks some other glands may get swollen but they are painless and easily escape notice. There is usually a patchy rash on part of the trunk or the upper parts of limbs and there are some pimply spots. Inside the mouth may be found some streaky red-margined tracks of greyish colour looking rather as if a garden snail had crawled there. They are called snail-track ulcers. And that may be all you'll see before the disease goes underground to infiltrate various parts of the body. From then on it is difficult to treat. So, if you are promiscuous or even occasionally sleep round, and if you notice the most insignificant pointers mentioned above, do get help at once.

Gonorrhoea is far less severe. Most cases fall into the trivial category unless there are complications. It too is caught by sexual contact during which a tiny germ called a coccus infects the moist lining of the urethra. Women can carry the germ while not having any symptoms themselves. Up to about thirty per cent of prostitutes carry the germ at least from time to time. Very rarely the disease is spread on fingers or on soiled towels or clothes. Like syphilis, it can affect the rectum after anal sex, or the mouth after oral sex. It too can eventually spread to joints, liver, heart and even brain if neglected. It is, however much easier and more effectively treated if caught early. Two to eight days after exposure there is a sudden onset of frequency, urgency, pain on passing water and a discharge of pus (all as in urethritis above). Sometimes there is no pain but if the prostate gland or seminal vesicles are affected, pain may be considerable and there may be a rise in temperature. The disease is often self-limiting, and may settle after a few weeks and without spreading. This cannot be relied on, however, and even after the disease is over the sufferer may remain a carrier or may have strictures (tiny bands of tight scar tissue) around the urethra kinking it or even closing it later in life.

**Special Section follows:-**

AIDS: (Acquired Immune Deficiency Syndrome) This is probably one of the greatest current threats to mankind. It is constantly worsening. At this time it seems likely that many will die.

What is AIDS?

It stands for Acquired Immune Deficiency Syndrome. A syndrome is nothing more that a group of symptoms and physical signs that can be grouped together as a recognisable clinical condition or diagnosis. Acquired means you got it or caught it somewhere rather than being born with it or developing it yourself. The human body is subjected, day in day out, to endless risks from outside influences ranging from chemical poisons to infectious bacteria. It therefore needs its resistance system comprised of an extremely complex and efficient collection of protective mechanisms. These prevent or combat the infecting organisms thereby rendering the person 'immune' to them. If this immune system is impaired or lacking in some way, it is spoken of as being deficient.

What do you catch?

You catch a chemical,.. of a kind. But it is a very special kind of chemical. It is a virus, which is a chemical which when it enters certain kinds of living hosts, behaves as if it too were in some way 'alive.' At first a mere few of the host's cells are infiltrated. Later this number may vastly increase. The health and function of the cells is generally curtailed and they may die. If a large number of the cells of a vital tissue or type die off, the general health of the host may no longer be sufficient for survival. Disease and even death will then follow unless the damaging trend can be reversed.

Because the virus that causes (or is, at least, closely associated with) AIDS affects the immune system cells of humans it is commonly called HIV. This does not mean, as many seem to think, 'H-4' in Roman numerals. It is the abbreviation for Human Immuno-Virus. Someone who is carrying the HIV is said to be 'HIV-Positive.'

What Happens Next?

Usually not very much for a while. In many cases, having entered some of the cells, the virus becomes dormant there. Though remaining alive and well, it doesn't proliferate and spread. This quiescent interval may last weeks, months or even years. While it continues the patient is spoken of as a carrier, but does not develop active disease. Unfortunately many are nevertheless infectious. If so, those who are ignorant of the time-bomb within them may well pass on their infection to lovers and loved-ones.

Eventually however, the virus is liable to become active and start to infiltrate more and more cells. The integrity of the essential cells of the protective immune system is often damaged beyond repair when the HIV takes up residence. The result of this is that the body is no longer properly screened from other invading organisms such as bacteria. These too start to enter and take hold. The more common organisms, by sheer weight of numbers, naturally tend to be the first to enter and in the largest numbers. Bacteria that normally live, fairly harmlessly, in the body, start to multiply, go out of control and cause symptoms. Some that are often to be found even on a healthy skin, penetrate into the hair follicles and set up infections there. The result is a series of spots or boils, small at first, but which increase in size and number until an entire crop of pus-discharging ulcers form. Bacteria in the mouth also invade the tissues and outbreaks of trench-mouth, streptococcal sore throats, or other forms of stomatitis become common. Abscesses develop in the ears. The eyes and nose, always harbouring bacteria from the environment, also become infected and purulent. Elsewhere the fingernails can become surrounded by whitlows. Bacteria from the bowels establish infections both there and in the neighbouring urinary bladder. The vagina too is easily exposed as is the male foreskin, both becoming the focus of serious and damaging infection.

Within the body other viruses and inhaled bacteria attack the lungs causing first dangerous inflammation and then pneumonia. Infections, over a period of weeks or months, often spill over into the bloodstream and the resulting septicaemia spreads the infection throughout the body including, with immense danger to life, to the kidneys, liver and brain.

The general ill-health causes anaemia, loss of appetite, pallor, weight-loss and profound weakness. The patient goes downhill, often rapidly, until the accumulating toxins and the utterly overwhelmed body resistance bring about total collapse and death.

Whatever the sequence, AIDS is here,.. and it is going to kill large numbers. It is an exceedingly glum picture.

Where is it now?

Official handouts are coy about the present high-risk areas. USA, Central Africa and Western Europe are danger spots. San Francisco and New York are highly infiltrated. Mexico has a twenty five per cent homosexual exposure. Other black spots are Haiti, St.Lucia and the Dominican Republic. In Uganda there is a growing twenty per cent infection rate and they expect a quarter of a million deaths in the next two years. In Nairobi the hotel-prostitute carrier rate is a horrifying ninety per cent.

In Europe the four worst affected countries are France, Germany, UK. and Italy, in that order. Two thirds of UK. cases are in London and the S.East. WHO experts estimated 50,000 carriers in the USA. alone in 1993 and an increase to around three million ten years from then, with one third progressing to actual AIDS. The exposure rate is doubling roughly annually.

These figures are really based on those issued,.. or leaked, some two or three years ago. Although highly alarming it is recognised everywhere that the figures have already been drastically exceeded.

How do you get it?
So far only one certain method is known. It is believed that AIDS can only be caught from another person. That other person must be either a carrier or actually suffering clinical symptoms. And contact needs to be very intimate. What has to happen is referred to as a transmission of body fluids. Theoretically this means anything fluid,.. urine, blood, faeces, saliva, semen. In effect however, it has to be a fluid in which there are active components of the HIV, usually in or from infected cells also present in the fluid.

This is not the only difficulty. Most viruses, and the HIV is one such, find the human skin to be an impenetrable barrier. They need an easier route. Direct access to the body via a wound is easiest for them. A second best is to be deposited somewhere on the mucous membrane, the wet, pink, 'inner skin' that lines body orifices like the mouth, rectum and vagina.

From this data, the methods of entry can be deduced. Blood from an infected person can be put directly into the blood of a patient receiving a transfusion. Many deaths already resulted from this before blood bank donors were adequately screened. Inadvertent exchange of blood is a disastrously common likelihood in the drug-taking communities. Seriously addicted junkies grow notoriously incautious with their hygiene measures. To them, the important thing is to get the next dose in as fast as possible. So, if a group is to share a supply, say of heroin, the same hypodermic syringe may well be used, passed from hand to hand. It is the perfect transmission weapon.

Semen is also a highly suitable medium for carrying HIV. The vaginal mucous membrane can be fairly easily penetrated especially if repeatedly exposed. However as, during its natural function, it is normally subjected to exposure from outside infections, it has a considerable protective resistance. The rectum is not similarly equipped as its penetration is not visualised in nature. Consequently male homosexual activities involving penetration of another male rectum are likely to result in the spread of HIV. Small wounds, cracks or fissures are common around both vaginal and rectal orifices as a result of other infections, scratching and so on. If present, these too vastly increase the chances of spread by providing a gap in the defences. The sexual route of transmission is therefore now available to male/male and male/female intercourse. Homosexuals in contact with the androgynous individuals (colloquially known as AC/DC) spread infections to them. They, in turn, may contact other males, 'free' females or their own long-term female partners. In this way heterosexual spread has much increased in recent years. It remains however, a less likely hazard.

Much research has been carried out on other methods of spread. Facts are few and data supplied is not always reliable. For example, unsterilised acupuncture needles are, like hypodermic needles, proven vehicles of transmission. Authorities, some of them medical, who disapprove of unorthodox medical techniques, have blamed this route as fervently as those who are members of the anti-drug lobby blame misuse of dirty syringes. Their fears are genuine if a shade disingenuous. But there have been political trade-offs. In return for weighty criticism of these two routes, many have kept silent about the at least equally great fear that could be incurred in the population in relation to insect transfer. It has long been known that some insect pests transmit blood-borne diseases. Some body lice transmit fevers,.. mosquitoes transmit malaria,.. and mosquitoes can thus, at least in theory, transfer the HIV from one of its hosts to the next.

And there is increasing certainty that the virus can remain active for surprisingly long periods even outside of a host. Virus spread by 'droplet infection' on the breath as with the common cold can also not be adequately excluded.

Further research has detected AIDS in the new-born infants of infected mothers. Other researchers are working on transmission via breast milk and even saliva. Organisational reassurance is, at the very least, suspect. Much is at stake and, currently, even the subsequent discovery of transmission via perspiration, say from one sweaty hand to another during handshake, is far from permanently excluded. The word is clear,.. take extreme caution.

What can you do about it?

The blunt truth is that once you have got it you can do nothing more than pray. Despite the investment of millions of dollars, man hours and high-tech, there is nothing, even on the distant horizon, that promises cure of those infected with HIV. The best hope is that, having infected someone, it may lie dormant for many years. Once it goes active however, death is a virtual certainty. And the death will usually be slow, insidious, degrading and painful. Patients face the sure, downward path through infections, debility and social ostracism until they die a wretched and painful death from wasting and weakness.

The reality is that current medical management centres around preventing spread,.. alleviating unpleasant symptoms though without any prospect of cure,.. and giving mental and physical support during the declining and dying stages.

No chemical or pharmaceutical agent yet produced has anything but a local or minimal effect. There is no curative antibiotic. There is no vaccine that protects. There is not even any great prospect of anything turning up soon. At present, the word cure does not even belong in the vocabulary!

The solution then, pro tem, does not depend upon cure. It relies totally on prevention. And prevention means avoiding contact of all kinds with all affected people. This raises a serious collision between the instinctive ostracism of society and the more humanitarian inclinations. Some parents have been reluctant to allow their children to attend schools where AIDS suffering children, or merely the so far uninfected children of known AIDS cases, are pupils. Many people are equally reluctant to frequent restaurants where waiters may be homosexual. Similarly in relation to contact with other areas where there tend to be substantial numbers of homosexuals,.. show business, hair dressers, haute couture and so on. There is no doubt that certain groups,.. junkies, black people and homosexuals have experienced a hardening of attitudes towards them, attributable to the AIDS risk. Each individual must decide personally where his or her line must be drawn between humanitarian motives and the sheer practicalities of living and the fear or risk of infection.

In some areas however, the danger is so great that there should be no hesitation in scrupulous avoidance. All forms of sexual contact that involve the exchange of body fluids should cease except with those partners known to be uninfected. The general precautions are now well-publicised. Don't have contact with junkies, or homosexuals. Don't get involved with promiscuous, easy-lay sex partners. Wash the genitals before and after sex. Always use a protective condom. Don't allow any part of the body with even a slight wound into sexual contact.

It is true that some individuals and organisations who are of anti-permissive views have sought to exaggerate the risks of heterosexual promiscuity. Nevertheless, these risks do exist. The extent is uncertain, to be sure, but it is great enough to merit extreme caution. The fact is that when you have sex with someone, as far as AIDS is concerned, you are also having sex with everyone they've had sex with for the last ten years. That's how long the HIV could have lain dormant in them. Before you do it then, be sure you want to run that kind of risk.

What of the future?

The future is very bleak and the overall situation is worsening rapidly. At present rates alone, within the early years of next century, one tenth of the population of the earth will probably be affected. And that is the good news!

We are at the start of a pandemic that makes the Black Death look like an outbreak of influenza. Yet, at this time, world governments are pussyfooting about and trying to save money, while being careful not to frighten anyone or, above all, not to offend anyone. In a crisis situation they are attempting to spare feelings.

Regrettably the present writer has nothing even remotely encouraging to say. One miserable little virus seems all set to achieve what centuries of gonorrhoea, syphilis, religion and social pressure between them could not. There must shortly follow either a drastic fall in promiscuity or a drastic fall in the population of the planet.

Final Comment: AIDS is, at present, such a dangerous disease and is spreading so virtually out of control everywhere, that all sexually active people should take all necessary protective precautions like wearing a condom for sex, all of the time. There are no exceptions.

**WARNING:** AIDS KILLS,.. horribly! It is rampant in our society. It is totally out of control. It is a very real and ever-present likelihood. It must *NOT* be underestimated. YOU CAN CATCH IT,.. easily!! You can spread it to your loved ones. They will probably die too. AIDS is the greatest-ever enemy of indiscriminate and promiscuous sexual habits. DON'T RISK IT!!

\* \* \*

For any kind of VD you should see a doctor. Most family doctors are understanding, kind and helpful. If not you can go straight to a Hospital Special Clinic or to a Board of Health Clinic. You don't usually even need an appointment. You can, if you prefer, even attend in a different town from where you live so no-one you know is likely to see you. If in doubt, do go anyway. It protects you, your loved ones and maybe your future children. And keep attending until follow-up tests conclusively show you are cured. Short cuts are stupid and so is home doctoring. Wearing a contraceptive sheath reduces the chances of infection for both partners. So does not leaving the penis in the vagina very long once orgasm has been accomplished. Antibiotics after a risky exposure might be worth considering as a preventive measure. The best bet is simply not to put your most priceless possession in a place where a sensible man would not put the ferrule of his umbrella. But if you must and do, take the precaution of using a condom properly. Make sure it fits. Put it on correctly. It has at least a 50% protection rate and in most cases, far higher. Spermicidal creams, diaphragms and sponges have an even greater protection rate in many conditions. Using a spermicide and a condom is the best disease preventing combination yet devised.

**Vasectomy:** This is not a disease but seems to fit better here than anywhere else. It is the name of the operation for male sterilisation. One or two half-inch cuts are made under local (injection) or general anaesthetic, into the skin of the scrotum. Each vas in turn is brought out through the hole, severed, and the hole stitched closed again with one or two small sutures which are painlessly removed a few days later. Apart from the pinprick of the injections the operation doesn't hurt at all. Afterwards the entire scrotum can feel pretty tender, often for a few days. If there is much internal bleeding it may also become bluish or bruised-looking though this scarcely increases the pain or soreness. Some operations that are now being developed are intended to be reversible; if it is wished the cut ends of the vas can then later be rejoined at another operation, thus restoring fertility. However, most operations are not of this type and at present should be regarded as permanent. [Make sure which you have if this matters to you]. There are no significant after-effects to be expected. Sperms are simply reabsorbed harmlessly into the body. The semen ejaculated looks and tastes just the same. There is nothing to fear from vasectomy. Above all it does not affect the libido or decrease the sexual performance, indeed, it may increase it. Under no conditions does it reduce that strange quality a man calls his 'manhood.' I've never been quite certain exactly what that is and no-one has ever succeeded in describing it to me, but I'm sure that wherever it lives, it is not in the vas and therefore survives the operation quite undamaged.

\* \* \*

**Chapter Ten:** Sex Faults of the Penis

Apart from the actual disease conditions discussed in the previous chapter, there are sexual disorders not of the genital organs themselves, but of the way they work. That means purely and simply where the causes are emotional rather than physical. If a man's penis won't work it is not usually its fault, it's his. If a woman's vagina hurts when a penis gets inside it, again it's not usually its fault, it's hers,.. or, perhaps his. Sexual dysfunctions or non-functions are a bit like accidents,.. they don't happen, they are caused. They are invariably due to mental hang-ups. These crippling results of wrong conditioning, prejudice, lazy thinking (or the total lack of it) or other peoples' behaviour are the cause of more human misery that perhaps any other factor. Yet incredibly little notice is taken of them, their understanding and their treatment either at personal or national level.

More or less everybody has a sexual problem at least once in a lifetime. It may be a brief episode for the lucky ones. For others it is long drawn out and can, for years, cloud every other aspect not only of their own lives but of those near to them at home, work and play.

**Life-styles and your sex-life**
The largest source of sexual problems is inflexibility. By this is meant rigidity of attitude. If ever the advice to 'loosen up' was good advice it is in relation to sex. Everything in life changes. Preferences for clothing styles, foods, drinks and motor cars all move steadily on throughout life (though certain detectable themes may be continuous). Sex is the same, or should be. Superimposed on the theme or pattern formulated by genetic and other factors, it should be a developing phenomenon. It may be the affectionate expanding repertoire of a couple happily related and adjusted for many years. All well and good if it is. But even outside of a stable relationship sex should be a phenomenon of continuously broadening knowledge and improving technique.

**Solving sexual problems**
The whole sexual mechanism is so complex and delicate that it is extremely vulnerable to influences from without. The cause of the trouble may be a tense working atmosphere or an anxious financial period. The cause may be an unsatisfactory degree of adjustment in a partnership. But nearly always the cause involves someone else. Commonly the fault will only exist with one person. A woman, set in her sexual habits, may be unaroused for years by her husband, but may respond in minutes in the hands of an unimportant lover. A man hung-up with jealousy may fail only with the object of his jealousy while he can masturbate with ease or succeed with another less worthy partner. Two things are sure. Almost any sexual problem that is caused can be improved and it is frequently someone else's help that does the improving.

One requirement is needed above all others in the treatment of sexual disorders. Since they are so frequently caused by under- or over- motivation, it is in the field of motivation that they are best tackled. If there is someone who doesn't want to improve and who really is satisfied (many just pretend to be for reasons they may not know even exist) then they are nothing but a liability. Without change there is no progress. Without progress there is only perpetual sameness. If someone is too slightly motivated to wish to help then that person is worthless as a genuine partner.

There are several programmes devised for combating the various sexual problems. These will now be discussed. Where further advice or details of such programmes are needed there are booklets available which can be used as instruction manuals. These are mentioned in the section on Sexual Aids in Chapter Eleven.

**Premature ejaculation**

The commonest sexual problem in younger men, this is usually thought of as a purely male problem. Broadened to the phrase *premature orgasm* however, it includes him and her. Much of what is said about him applies to her equally. Premature orgasm is any orgasm that happens before both want it to. For some couples, for example, simultaneous orgasm, both reaching the peak together, is the ultimate sexual aim. Indeed, for most couples it is the aim at least sometimes. However, the techniques used on another occasion may be such that the climaxes are deliberately separated, one partner bringing the other to orgasm first. Either way if the peak comes too soon it spoils other things. So it is premature. The man or woman who is able to enjoy more than one orgasm (and as we shall see it is largely a matter of training), is untroubled by an occasional premature climax. That in itself is one good reason for training. But it is on training that the treatment of premature ejaculation also depends.

The usual complaint is from him. (Probably over ninety per cent of premature orgasms are male). The description is relentlessly similar in so many instances. He is normally aroused. His penis assumes its largest proportions. Then, before he is ready, and quite without his control, he ejaculates. Sometimes this is into her hand or mouth, sometimes over the bedclothes. Most frequently of all though, it is as he brings his penis against her vulva or during its first strokes inside her. Just when she is anticipating her penetration, he comes, and at once goes too soft to be of any value. As a rule, the problem for her is less. By fortunate coincidence the large majority of premature orgasms in women occur in those who, although they may not have achieved the step yet, are potentially multi-orgasmic types. On questioning they often at first deny this, but closely pressed they can usually recall rare occasions when they had three or four orgasms within a quarter of an hour. The same is not true for him. He ejaculates once and finds the proceedings are over at least for a while. His penis may even for some minutes prove uncomfortable to touch.

Here at once is one of the first lines of treatment. Instead of giving up he should try a brief pause (ten minutes is plenty) then try starting again. There is no doubt in my experience that it is the active participation by her in using her skills and especially her knowledge of him that brings the biggest success rate by this method. An alternative is for him to masturbate a while beforehand. By taking the edge off his eagerness, when it comes to the real thing he performs better. Another approach, after orgasm, is for him to await his next erection by entering her from behind, while both lie on their sides. Quite a soft penis will enter in this way and as soon as down in the forest something stirs, it's time for further action. The treatment should start early as premature ejaculation can become a nervous habit like nail biting if it goes on too long. Long established cases are harder to cure.

If such simple measures have not succeeded, more effort is required. Sooner or later after his orgasm he recharges and is able to erect again. When he has done so, both should aim to hold him back by keeping stimulation to a minimum. The aim is to stay rigid as long as possible without an orgasm. It needs to be practised frequently to be effective. After a time it should be possible to increase stimulation even to the extent of keeping the penis in her mouth or vagina without ejaculation. This is similar to the *karezza* technique in which the penis is kept in the vagina without movement in order to prolong intercourse or prevent ejaculation or both.

**The 'stop' method**
For resistant cases a more radical technique is nearly always effective. He waits until he feels orgasm approach. It does not matter whether this is with the penis already in the vagina or prior to that stage. Whenever orgasm approaches, that is the moment. Well before it happens,.. and timing is crucial,.. he says, "Stop." When he says it she does it. Whatever stage things are, all movement ceases. This is often enough. When tension falls the action resumes, gently. The process is repeated several times before orgasm is allowed to be completed.

For those in whom it proves impossible to penetrate the vagina before a premature ejaculation happens, things can be taken further. She should masturbate him by hand only. When he calls the halt, she not only stops but grips his glans between her finger and thumb and squeezes it hard enough to cause actual slight discomfort. This is not dangerous but will quell any but the most insistent ejaculation. (Note: it doesn't matter if he ejaculates while she is holding the aperture shut, but it may be uncomfortable).

If this stage is reached while the penis is actually deep within the vagina, the glans is not accessible to her. Instead she should reach down and grasp his testicles firmly in her hand and apply some pressure to them. They should practice this beforehand. That way he can tell her how hard she can or should squeeze to cause the necessary discomfort but without producing real pain.

This entire technique of learning and practising the 'stop' method is the correct approach for her too if she wishes to delay her orgasm. She should masturbate for as long as she can, then exert her will power and discontinue when she gets near her climax. If she goes too far she presses hard on her clitoris, or if it is large enough, grips and squeezes it until sensation subsides. Later on she can have him masturbate her until the 'stop' moment. Later still, during intercourse, the technique remains the same. If she gets too close he stops all movements and one or other applies pressure to some part of the her genital zone for a few moments. He should leave enough gap between his body and hers to ensure this is possible.

If a couple repeatedly fail to orgasm, separately or together, more or less always at the time of their choosing, it will usually be found that one or other is far more seriously afflicted. Either way control can and should be learned. It is one of the foundation stones of relationship adjustment. If you cannot control timing you cannot successfully develop different techniques. Anyone can learn and, as with most things, practice makes perfect.

**Impotence**
Probably the most common disease throughout all of Western society today is sexual impotence. It is also the cause of the greatest fear. For if ever there is a word or an idea that strikes terror into a man, it is impotence. Yet the fears are largely irrational. As we shall see, the causes are such that most can be avoided, many resisted, and plenty overcome.

Impotence exists in a number of degrees. There may be complete or partial inability to gain an erection when it is wanted. Or the inability may be not so much to gain an erection but to maintain it for as long as it is wanted. There may be total failure to achieve ejaculation as a natural conclusion to a sexual encounter. The biggest trouble with impotence is that it cannot be hidden. A woman who has been unable to achieve sexual arousal or satisfaction can pretend otherwise. Some do. Some can't be bothered. But the impotent male can do nothing to conceal his inability. The evidence of what he feels to be the very essence of his manhood, his utter sexual weakness and inability, is exposed to ridicule before the very person or persons from whom he would most of all wish it kept a secret. The effect upon him is incalculable. His entire self-image and ego-product is deflated. He sees himself humiliated in the eyes of himself and others. This is not only a bad enough situation in itself for its disastrous ability to reduce confidence and respect, but it can initiate a series of other symptoms that are even worse. A man's efforts to compensate can be so terrible if successful, and so destructive if not, that it is hard to know which is worse.

Much of the trouble arises from ignorance. The whole question of impotence has been surrounded by ridiculous myths. Actual knowledge is very limited. As a result, a lot of false deduction and gibberish has been substituted. Common sense would have been far better. Nowadays we have reached the stage of making sick but very realistic jokes like, "What's the difference between anxiety and fear? Anxiety is the first time you can't do it the second time; fear is the second time you can't do it the first time."

**Impotence facts**
Virtually every man (and woman) gets occasional impotence and it is of no significance. If only men realised that when it happens to them they are just temporary members of a huge club and that on their way to the office they will probably pass a dozen others similarly affected, it is a great help. The nonsensical concept that a man is a rampant sex demon filled to overflowing with repeated orgasms and floods of semen as ever-ready as a torch battery is simply not true. His sexuality may be built-in, but it needs servicing and attention if it is to work smoothly. It can go wrong easily enough.

One of the ways the temporarily impotent man can gain reassurance is to try masturbating alone. It often works thus proving his machinery is intact. Or, he may discover at night or in the early morning that he has an unintended erection (the so-called 'three-quarter stand' or 'morning wood'). This too shows that his mechanism still works. He can therefore look forward to a considerable measure of ultimate success. Worrying is a great worsener and never makes him better.

Physical causes of impotence exist in plenty. For example, many diseases cause or predispose to it. About 40% of all impotence cases reported are due to medication. The true proportion including all cases can only be estimated but is probably rather a lower figure. Diabetics are particularly prone to periods of impotence. So are people who are overweight. So are people on some kinds of blood pressure treatments. So are people who drink and smoke too much. Already, though, these latter 'physical' causes can be seen to be in those of fragile emotional dispositions. Otherwise they wouldn't need to drink, smoke or get overweight.

Although often blamed, age alone is not the greatest cause of impotence. Ease of arousal and frequency of arousal do both decrease with years. The main significance of age is that as it brings greater experience and familiarity, it can also mean that in sex, as in many other things, people need greater levels of stimulation, physical, visual, mental and so on to get the same result. Sexually this results in a natural inclination towards expansion of techniques and outlets. Mostly what the older person needs is more direct and indirect stimulation. Given this, neither male more female potency should be much affected until well on into the later decades. A frequent complaint from women is the way that age makes them less attractive while their menfolk commonly get more so. Women however have an immense ability to compensate. It is mainly during her forties that a woman reaches the level of emancipation and understanding that frees her from her old inhibitions. At last she starts to acquire techniques which make her more than ever before precious to the sexually aware man. At last she starts to enjoy sex. She needs only to put as much time into practising sex as into reading her glossy magazines to achieve a sexuality that would previously have astonished her. Her man will seldom go out looking for what he can find at home.

**The psychology of impotence**

So to the psychological causes of impotence. These are of two main types that we may call performance fears and sexual hang-ups. Performance fears tend to arise only occasionally, usually on special occasions. For example, after a long absence a man may be sexually frustrated and over-excited at the idea of his first night back with his wife. He expects too much of himself and the situation. Sadly she may misinterpret his failure as having been caused by recent infidelity. Or he may have drunk too much at a wedding anniversary dinner. Or she might put him off by being fractious and quarrelsome for a similar reason. Wedding nights are a shocking example. To expect an inexperienced couple, after a hectic and exciting day, too much to drink and perhaps a long journey, to go to bed and perform a complicated sexual act just right first time is unrealistic. Ideally there should be a lot of planning, including intercourse, long before that stage. The experienced approach to sexual encounters is the one that pays. Calculated indifference or careful nonchalance often succeeds in overcoming impotence and is worth encouraging. The story of the young bull and the old bull who spotted some attractive cows in a field explains the point. The young bull said, "Let's you and me rush over there and screw a couple of those cows." The old bull said "No. Let's you and me stroll over there and screw the lot."

The biggest of all groups by far is that of sexual hang-ups,... the mental blocks and inhibitions. These always result from wrong conclusions either in the sufferer, his partner, or both. Most men or women who are impotent are so because they are up against a sexual hang-up of their own or their partner's that they are finding it hard to overcome. These were usually developed earlier in life because of the endless clash between the enormous power of the sex drive and the way it has been curtailed and made a taboo subject of disgust and even sin by foolish societal impositions. The stupidity and ignorance of teachers, religionists, equally confused parents and so on have combined to distort the true, decent, beautiful and natural context of sexual acts.

Fortunately nowadays inhibitions can be recognised, classified, understood and adjusted so they need not comprise any reason for fear. A woman can become frigid if her man lets her stimulation and satisfaction level fall too low or if he gives her no feedback on her efforts to please him. Her confidence subsides below threshold level. A man or woman can become impotent if made to feel guilty because of a deviation they possess.

Self-protective phenomena like jealousy, infidelity, criticism, ridicule and callousness of approach always make things worse. There are endless ways in which those twin spectres of selfishness and misunderstanding can get into headlong top gear. Impotence becomes ingrained. The relationship is on the rocks.

**The treatment of impotence**

This book is not the right place in which to give a detailed description of impotence therapy. There are other, more extensive books such as that on the 'Twenty Minute Miracle Method,' a selection of which have been listed for that purpose in the Sources List at the end of this book. But impotence is so important and so common, that a few brief words of explanation and guidance cannot be excluded.

It is now clear that both treatment and cure of impotence are entirely feasible. The main prong of attack is speed. It is imperative to get to the root of the trouble swiftly and then make an all-out effort. No effort is too great or too soon. Both partners must be involved, deeply. There are things each can do.

His first job is to improve his general physical health. Partly this is because good health is physically conducive to potency, partly because there is a corresponding increase in personal pride which helps immensely on a psychological level. He should consult a good set of height-weight tables and start getting his weight down to the correct level. The chances are he should reduce his consumption of alcohol,.. never more than two pints of beer or three shots of spirit a day; and cigarettes,.. never more than five a day. He probably needs more exercise. A good way is to walk at least two miles twice a week. He should go to bed at sensible hours, even if he reads while he is there. In all, it amounts to doing the simple things doctors always tell patients, to improve general condition. Two weeks is all he needs to start it working.

There are some male hormones that help sexual performance. (Funnily enough it is also the male hormone that influences female libido). Given in short sharp doses they may help to jolt the machinery into action. After any length of time though, they tend to cut down the body's own hormone manufacturing system, so they must stop. Some anxiety-reducing medication can sometimes be of value. Further help can come from the use of certain sexual aids as covered in greater detail in the next chapter.

An excellent way of improving erection and increasing general health and confidence at the same time is by using personal autohypnosis tapes. In the Sources List are detailed individual tapes made by experienced physicians rather than the usual hacks and quacks.

And what can she do to help? Well, undoubtedly her first value is in actual prevention. She should ensure that her attitude to sex is a healthy one. If she is a product of a bygone age when women were conditioned and forced into suppressing their sexuality under the pretence that their sex-drive is less than a man's (which it is not) she needs to revise her ideas. Reading a good book on sex should help. (See Sources List). She will almost certainly benefit from a course of libido training. There is a booklet containing a programme for that too mentioned later. Once her understanding of sex is that it is clean, respectable and enjoyable she should aim to take an active part in it. Both partners' aims should be to help each other by words and deeds from hand, mouth and mind. Make a practice of sitting and talking about sex. Discuss each other's likes and dislikes. Go further, delve for the reasons for them. Try to become the repository of each other's secret fantasies. Never use information so obtained in subsequent rows,.. its dirty fighting. Repeatedly go over problems and differences from every possible angle, dismantling fragment by fragment even if it causes friction. No cupboard gets a thorough airing by having its doors kept shut. Nothing was ever truer than that a trouble shared is a trouble halved. Look for hang-ups that you either have or cause. Encourage each others deviations. Develop pride in being sexy,.. it's natural after all, and highly unnatural to be unsexy. If she likes her toes sucked, suck them. If he likes black stockings, wear them. Above all, never be afraid to say you're sorry,.. sometimes even if you're not quite. It's never a sign of weakness.

By these efforts many cases of impotence will already be resolved. But what of those that are not? This is the place that she really comes into her own. She and she alone will hold the answer. In the name of love if she has it, and in the name of common decency even if she doesn't, it's her job. Her object should be the exact opposite to the role she plays in treating premature orgasm. This is the time to use every known ancillary aid to stimulation that she can find. Now is the time to be ready, willing and able. She should aim to turn herself into whatever he wants. No half measures or hanging back. She should use every trick in the book. She must dress right, talk right, act right, excite and be prepared to play sex games at every and any time - BUT - the action must stop short of orgasm. This is an essential pre-requisite and must be firmly decided by both in advance. He must know that whatever happens he is not expected to orgasm or make her orgasm. Nothing is to be expected of him. With his anxiety and tension thus reduced, his suspicions allayed, he is subjected to her overwhelming efforts at excitement. Chakravarti mentions the great value of the new and different sensation of completely shaving the pubis, testicles, vaginal lips and around the anus. Above all be patient and keep trying. Drs.Masters and Johnson (whose names should go down in the sexual role of honour) have shown conclusively that it can be done. Modern development of their original 'Sensate Focus' technique are now effectively used everywhere. If you need this purchase a good programme booklet and start re-training. Or read *'Impotence,... and its Home Treatment by the Twenty Minute Miracle Method.'* (See Sources List). This is a recent book which details a remarkable short cut which few realise exists. Its success rate has been good enough to make it eminently worth a try. The technique was first proposed by an American physician. It consists of a simplified programme for the busy, troubled man. After briefly explaining impotence there is a first class list of possible causes. Yours may be amongst them. If it is your problem may be solved in less than twenty minutes! If not, the technique of success via Sensate Focus is explained. This method guarantees a sexual encounter, limited perhaps, but with the certainty of penetration within the first twenty minutes of the correct stage being reached. This alone makes it remarkable,.. and at least in part thoroughly justifies the word 'miracle.'

An American device, also marketed in UK. and Europe and designed to assist erection is the Post-T-Vac vacuum therapy. It consists basically of a suction device to fit over the penis and a suitable range of adapters and constriction rings to maintain the erection achieved. It also has a built-in pressure gauge for monitoring suction/evacuation. Post-T-Vac is ethically marketed as an erection device only. Regrettably its price is substantially higher at around £250 ($400).

Yet another aid to erection is the ErecAid also available in a number of countries. Less complex and less costly than Post-T-Vac the principle is similar. A grip operated suction device enables partial erection which is then encircled by an elastic band-type of constrictor ring.

The similarity of these methods to the Penatone siphon was noted by the Editorial Consultant of the British Journal of Sexual Medicine. In this writer's opinion Penatone remains the best all-round method of penis enhancement as it is the only ethical-medical programme to aim not only at erection but at developing and increasing penis size, sensitivity and performance all at the same time. It is detailed later.

Other impotence treatments include surgical implantation of stiffening devices actually into the penis. In correctly chosen cases results are good. The devices may be semi-rigid, flexible, or 'inflatable' from a fluid reservoir usually concealed within the scrotum. These methods have, in recent years, been overtaken by two forms of pharmaceutical help that have revolutionised impotence therapy especially for cases of psychological origin. In one of these an active substance is either injected directly into the shaft of the penis immediately before sex or is inserted, as a tiny tablet into the meatal end of the urethra via the 'eye' of the penis head. These chemicals have the effect of increasing blood supply and therefore erection. They are very effective indeed though many men dislike the use of injections into the penis. Most popular of all is the arrival of the new compounds [Viagra and similar] which can be equally effective when taken by mouth in tablet form about half an hour to an hour before sex is intended.

**The Sex Magnetrode**
In recent years vast amounts of research have begun to discover the value of magnetism for numerous therapeutic purposes. It is now used to improve circulation, to hasten bone healing, for full-body resonance, for reducing the pain and inflamation of rheumatism and arthritis and so on. One snag has been the expense of powerful magnetic devices. Many other projects are nevertheless in the experimental stage now that mass production has started to reduce costs so drastically. All this has caused those working in Sexual Medicine to reconsider the possible values of magnetism in their field too,.. values that had hitherto been laughed off as ridiculous.

The result has been the production of the Sex Magnetrode. This is a powerfully induced and balanced magnetic field producer. Although it sounds complex it is merely a small disc of active metal surrounded by a simple plastic shield. The Magnetrode is kept, unobserved, in the trousers pocket and is, from there, able to contain the genital zone within a field that most find to be rapidly beneficial. Enthusiasts wear one in each pocket to double the effect!

Ladies use them too, also in pockets, or tucked into waist-bands where influence can be projected towards their ovaries and genitals. Not surprisingly, users have also reported other than merely sexual effects particularly on their daily aches, pains and screws. Magnetrodes can be recommended for trial by anyone as their success rate is very high indeed.

**A magical extra**
There is another excellent pharmaceutical product that should be tried by every sufferer from impotence, slight or severe,.. and indeed by everyone wishing to ensure the highest sexual fitness and performance levels.

Suppositories,.. for self administered rectal insertion, exist to improve the sexual systems of both men and women. They rely on sound medical principles, using the immune system to tone up and improve the function of all the tissues involved in sexual activity. Unfortunately the suppositories are in short supply and there is only one medical supplier in UK. There has not yet been time for submission to the United States FDA so they are not yet obtainable there at all though they can, of course, be perfectly legally ordered from England (See Sources List). Both preparations were developed by physicians specialising in sexual medicine in Europe and it is no wonder that they are the treatments most widely used by doctors on themselves,.. and their wives. Called Masculone and Feminone, a course of these suppositories belong in the bathroom cupboard of every sexually active person, man or woman, once or twice a year.

\* \* \*

So, most sexual problems live in the mind and are caused by the mind,.. your own or someone else's. It is everyone's duty to help his or her partner by understanding and going along. Sex is good, clean, healthy and progressive fun. The more of it you have the better you will be. Remember, the actual time spent at sex may involve less than an hour a week,.. a mere half of one per cent of your time. That is less time than it would take to smoke twenty cigarettes. Yet its value is out of all proportion. Anyone who spends more time thinking of smoking than of fucking and anyone who spends more time smoking than actually fucking just has to have got the priorities all wrong. The return on time spent on sex is the most profitable of all. So make a good and thorough job of the time you get. Sex can be the best thing there is and it's still free. Be prepared to drop anything, anywhere, any time, for sex.

\* \* \*

## Chapter Eleven: Sexual Aids

Sexual aids may be described as devices designed other than by nature to increase enjoyment of and performance in sexual behaviour. As such they can be used, by those in need, to correct a variety of sexual faults. Their main value to others is pleasure alone in that they widen the available sexual repertoire.

Now, whatever the relationship between a man and a woman, it has its foundation in sex. It may well be argued that a relationship or a marriage is made in Heaven. But it is certain that it will be preserved or otherwise in bed. And bed is by no means always heaven. Some naturally polygamous animals, and like it or not man is one of these, are able to form single, lasting, monogamous relationships. But these involve some deviation from the basic biological impulses and a devotion to other things than pure self. Because of this, such relationships are very vulnerable and nowhere more so than in bed.

### Overcoming boredom in your sex life

Whatever is your favourite kind of food you would soon tire of it three times a day and every day. This is especially so if you always eat it from the same plate, at the same time, at the same table and even wearing the same clothes. (One wit defined monotony as the state if being married to only one woman at a time). Many people are inhibited in their sex lives. They never learned much about it that was helpful. They perhaps never met anyone who gave them any enlightened experience. In spite of the so-called permissive society, for them sex is a dull, unimaginative routine. Pyjamas down and nighties up in a cold, dark, bedroom on a Saturday night after a tummy full of TV dinners and beer. Small wonder that they become bored and tired of all sex in general and of their partner's variety in particular.

Make no mistake, it is not just the ordinary man in the street who suffers. Couples in the very upper crust of society have just as many problems, though they do tend to be a somewhat different variety of problems. For all their education and incomes, they are as vulnerable as anyone else on the sensitive and easily upset balance of their sex lives. Even if they are mature and otherwise lovingly well-adjusted they can be disastrously affected.

### The bald penis

A couple of that very category will serve as an example. They arrived at the Sex Council Clinic in an expensive sports car. He was aged forty two, tall, well dressed and handsome. She was four years younger, a very beautiful blonde woman with smart clothes and a superb tan. They were a lucky couple. Not because they had a sexual problem, but lucky because they had found one of the few places where experts in sexual medicine work. They were lucky too because their own family doctor had recognised and appreciated their problem and had known where to send them. Lucky, most of all, because they were going to be cured.

Their story, when they got into conversation with the doctor, was that they had been happily married for twelve years. They had two children aged seven and ten and they had had, hitherto, a highly satisfactory sex life. Now, for the past several months, their sexual pleasures had been ruined because the wife was failing to orgasm. Their average number of sex acts was about three a week. The wife, when asked if she still enjoyed sex, answered, "Very much. Sometimes I look forward to it all day. I just can't wait for him to get home and when we do it it's lovely all the way through except that I jump about and try everything, but at the very end I don't seem to be quite able to make it anymore."

In a case like this a sensible couple would not have been alarmed by an occasional failure. It happens to everyone. But once fear and anxiety do start to rear their ugly heads they very quickly worsen a sensitive emotional situation.

Further questioning of our couple by their doctor disclosed the fact that the couple had for about six months been experimenting with something they had read about,.. the shaving off of the genital hair. They had found it exciting to shave each other there with the use of a small lady's electric shaver. The reason for starting this, they said, was because they had taken up going to judo classes and the protective boxes worn by some for the sport became entangled in and pulled at the pubic hair.

Being an expert, the doctor accepted their story but was convinced that the real motive was voyeurism. Not only did they enjoy shaving each other but they liked to see each other's sex organs so completely naked. They later agreed this was so. Furthermore, they said they had a number of mirrors in their bedroom.

And there lay the answer to their problem. During intercourse the crisp and curly male hairs stick out more than ever. They rub against the clitoris and surrounding area and assist in stimulating it. Now that the hair was gone the sensation was just not enough to take her over the top. The doctor prescribed a sexual aid of suitable type (which we shall be discussing later) and explained its use. The couple tried the treatment and it worked. It was a simple as that.

Clearly, if there are such simple ways of setting right problems that have a chance of spoiling happiness, even of threatening relationships, then it is in the interest of all to know about them. Surprisingly enough, this thought is by no means new. For sexual aids of one kind and another have been known and used in many places throughout history.

**Ancient sexual devices**
Even prehistoric man may have had his problems. Certainly we know that stones smoothed to resemble a penis were worn around the neck as ornaments. So were other stones with a smooth hole through them representing the vagina. It has been suggested that the stones may have been used in ritual religious coupling rites. But if some early rock paintings are correctly interpreted, the phallic stones were also used for insertion into the female. The holed stones were for masturbation by the men and were even sometimes worn around the penis during intercourse. As we shall see, many of today's sexual aids are similarly used.

In ancient Japan articles of clothing worn by the men were such that they had elaborately filled and projecting seams. These were grouped around the front of the thighs and around the root of the penis. During intercourse, for which clothing was not customarily removed, they would produce a great deal of friction over the female abdomen, thighs and buttocks. The Japanese are credited too with an invention for use by their womenfolk which is like today's vaginal strengthener (see later). Known by the name of ben-wa, the women got pleasure from wearing them internally and also developed the ability of their sexual muscles as a result. The beautiful paintings of the Chinese, such as the Golden Lotus, depicts such elaborate sexual aids as suspending a woman from a branch of a tree in a swing. The male lay precisely positioned beneath her while a servant gently swung the branch up and down.

From Arabic history also come examples of the ingenious use of articles as sexual aids. The techniques of producing sexual delight by softly rubbing both male and female organs with ripe peaches are well known. So is the idea of having intercourse actually through a large soft fruit. The travels of the explorer Sir Richard Burton and his elaborate writings on sexual subjects are another source of information about the use of sex aids in history. He tells, for example, of the habit of winding a stout cord around the root of the penis to enable a man not only to attain a bigger erection, but to maintain it for a longer time.

Coming closer to our own day, during the 1920's and 30's, a well-known firm of surgical instrument manufacturers of the highest ethical standing produced in England a range of artificial penises for issue mainly to men who had literally been dismembered during the carnage of the First World War. It was around this time too that there appeared the spreading knowledge of a gadget known ever since as the 'French Tickler.' This was a form of condom or sheath for the penis, from which small projections stood out and were designed to tickle or otherwise stimulate the vagina to greater pleasure during intercourse. At about the same time too Dr. Blakoe, also working in England, invented his famous Energising Ring, one of the most important sexual devices ever devised and of which we shall hear more later on in this book.

Throughout history then, sexual aids of one kind or another have been employed by both sexes. Great ingenuity has been displayed. The number of objects used as sexual aids by women has been incredible. (Nowadays, the variety of objects surgically removed from the vagina and urethra after being 'mislaid' during sexual use includes potatoes, cucumbers, bananas, bottles, doorknobs, paperclips and even corn cobs). Perhaps the best known of all examples of a sexual aid though is to be found in the Bible. There in Ezekiel, Chapter 16, verse 17, the prophet likens Jerusalem to an evil woman and admonishes her for the use of what is clearly a very expensive artificial penis.

In recent times the cheap and sordid sex shops of the late 1960's and 70's did much to ruin the image of the sex aid. Wanton profiteering, snide advertising and seedy premises and practices all helped to produce a false and damaging image. Aids began to be seen as something dirty, wicked and underhanded. Nothing could be further from the truth. The historically time-honoured value of sexual aids has not changed at all. Only two things are different. One is that modern scientific and medical interest has resulted in superior design which modern technology can better manufacture. The other is that with the increased freedom to discuss and enjoy sex both verbally and in print, there has come a wider knowledge and hopefully a more intelligent outlook. Over the years learned articles on the use of sex aids have appeared in all of the better medical journals from World Medicine to Pulse and the British Journal of Sexual Medicine. Doctors are learning too, and as long ago as 1975 perhaps the most famous medical school in Great Britain held a post-graduate symposium on sexual problems at which one of the three main papers, delivered by the present writer, was on Sexual Aids. There is no doubt that at long last they really have come to stay.

**The battle of the sexes**
One of the principle stumbling blocks to a successful sexual relationship is the basic differing sexual make-up of the male and female human being. Much has been made of the differences to be sure, and much exaggeration and distortion has crept in. The differences tend to have been artificially polarised, separated to their extremes and then

repeatedly conditioned into a pattern of acceptance so familiar as to pass virtually unquestioned. Somehow the idea of the woman as a domesticated creature dedicated to the kitchen and the maternal tasks of home-making has become associated with sexual disinterest and frigidity. The man, on the other hand, is seen as the virile breadwinner with a predatory and ever-ready sexual inclination. This view, while having a measure of truth, is by no means an entirely reliable and accurate assessment of the real state of affairs.

Normal males, as we all know, are sexually very easily aroused. They can achieve sexual readiness in the form of an erection sometimes in mere seconds and as a result of the slightest of excitement, perhaps only visual. They are physically able to copulate with almost any attractive female without hesitation and can proceed to orgasm and ejaculation within a minute or so. They may, of course, prefer to be more selective and to take their time. But they are equipped by nature to respond and perform in the manner described.

To an extent women differ. They are much more selective in their choice of males. They are less easily aroused except in the actual presence of the male. Their arousal too is less easy to initiate, and they usually need more time and attention to bring them to readiness for penetration. Even more prolonged periods of intercourse may be needed for them to orgasm.

These are the two main differences that cause the trouble. The female is slower to arouse in the initial stages and, partly as a consequence of this, her overall sexual requirements tend to average a lower frequency of encounters than the male, and she prefers a sustained period of intercourse for full gratification. All too commonly the male is over-insistent, over-frequent, over-clumsy and over too soon. The woman is unsatisfied, even annoyed or repelled. These are the factors that, together, comprise sexual dissonance,.. the discrepancy between male and female needs in terms of frequency and activities. If that sort of start to a relationship is allowed to continue, it easily deteriorates into a situation where the woman is described as frigid, the man as sex-mad and the relationship as incompatible.

**Women's lib and the sexual backlash**
One of the hidden and less desirable aspects of sexual freedom in recent years has come from the recognition by a growing number of women that sex can be very enjoyable. Not that that is a bad thing. Far from it. But it has meant that women have come to expect more from their partners. And the men have not always been up to it. While women were prepared to accept their age-old role of sexual inferiors, men could affect an air of experience while the women knew too little to prove them wrong. The new generation however, is coming to expect sexual fulfilment as surely as their menfolk. And why not indeed?

Oddly enough, instead of always pleasing them, this has caused an increase in the problems of a number of men. Some males have become anxious about their ability to satisfy. This is reflected in a gradual withdrawal from sex and a lowering in sexual esteem. The whole picture is one of great complexity but, against the background of today's pace of life and countless other problems, sex has retained its position at the top of the league of causes of unhappiness and illness.

Today in his consulting room the doctor sees a vast number of cases the origin of which is in psychological or emotional disturbances. Exact figures are hard to find, but the proportion has been estimated as between 20 per cent and 70 per cent of all the cases he sees. When the sexual appetite, titillated by the numerous aperitifs of modern living, is unsatisfied, malnutrition tends to manifest itself in many ways. "I keep getting these awful headaches, Doctor,.. this persistent skin rash,.. I never get a good night's sleep,.. I seem to cough and cough." These are phrases of everyday occurrence, as any doctor will tell. If he digs a little deeper he will soon uncover signs that his patients are sexually ill-adjusted. "Oh he's never satisfied,.. she's very good really, never says no,.. he's not so bad, Doctor, he doesn't bother me much." What a sad tale these remarks tell. They are all that shows of a dull, unhappy, unrewarding sex life. Yet, sex as was pointed out earlier, is the foundation of the relationship. If the foundation is not right, then nothing built upon that foundation can ever be right.

The problem is two-fold. There is the search for variety that is in the very nature of mankind. There is the need to overcome sexual problems like frigidity and failure to orgasm in the woman and impotence or premature ejaculation in the male. In these days of sexual freedom it has become all too easy to satisfy the need for change by promiscuous behaviour. But that still has always had many disadvantages,.. cost, organisation, fatigue, anxiety and the threat to a stable relationship for example. To that must now be added the overwhelmingly important reason of AIDS. Many, however, will prefer to find their variety with the same deeply loved mate. This is a theme around which an entire sexual programme can be developed, especially so in those over the age of about forty years. The entire subject and the kind of advanced sex that can be practised in such experienced couples is fully explained in the book, Age and Sex, mentioned in the Bibliography and Sources Lists. It should be regarded as essential reading by all serious students and practitioners of the sexual arts.

**Sexual aids and you**

When I lecture on the subject of Sexual Aids I normally begin by saying that I am not going to explain how listeners can pull sexual satisfaction out of their back pockets with the small change. The intention is to make an introduction to the use, and indeed, the very existence of sexual aids and to suggest how they might help in many sexual disorders. The same applies here.

Sexual aids do not cure all problems. Chronic sexual maladjustment needs more radical treatment. But, just as more headaches are treated by aspirins than by brain surgery, so many sexual disorders will respond to the correct choice and swift employment of a sexual aid.

The aids themselves fall naturally into two groups. Those to aid the female and those to aid the male. Many aid both partners simultaneously. When we consider female aids, it is as well to start at the beginning. The very first sexual problem in the female is that of the tight opening of the vaginal orifice in the virgin. In many ways this is paralleled later on in life by the condition called vaginismus. In this, usually for psychological reasons, the muscles of the vagina, especially around its opening, are kept very much contracted. This has the effect of partly closing off the approach to the vagina. When an attempt is made to penetrate with the penis, which may be as thick as say three fingers, it is so painful as to make it impossible. Indeed, sometimes it is so tight and the imagined or exaggerated idea of pain is so great that not even one finger tip can be inserted without howls and tears. Whether the cause is an emotional upset in an older woman or the naturally unstretched muscles of a teen-age virgin, the result is the same. It hurts to put anything in the vagina.

Particularly in relation to adolescent girls we have here a most unusual situation. We all know that early intercourse is usually painful. We all know that sooner or later most girls will go through this experience. We all know that clumsiness, inexperience and excitement can result in a loss of virginity that is looked back on in horror and which can give rise to sexual problems for the rest of a girl's life. And yet we do absolutely nothing about it. Although we know better,.. we neither help nor advise. The only word for that state of affairs is disgraceful.

**The friendly vibrator**

Nevertheless, in both the virgin and the vaginismus case there is help to be had; help which is almost always successful. For a start a girl can be taught how to practise gently on herself with her finger. Or we can recommend the use of one of today's most widely sold sexual aids, the vibrator. A vibrator consists of a tapering cylinder of plastic about six inches long and a little over an inch wide. Inside it is a small electric motor powered by batteries. The whole thing is harmless to use and easy to clean by rinsing with warm water and soap. At one end the cap which opens to admit the batteries, when closed and given an extra half turn, switches on the motor. This causes a small, heavy, off-centred weight in the middle of the vibrator to spin around. It is this oscillation which causes the actual vibration. There is no way that it can cause any kind of electric shock.

Some vibrators, while having all these usual basic aspects of construction, are very much more elaborate. For example, some are black. Some have a variety of interchangeable ends of different shapes and sizes. Some have a little illuminated tip. Some have a small control box. By turning the control knob the vibrations can be made faster and slower or more or less intense at will. Most elegant and not surprisingly the most popular of all today is one which not only vibrates in the ordinary way but also goes in and out.

The vibrator then is a prime example of a sexual aid that is not only of medical value but also, to many people, a lot of fun to use either personally for private masturbation or as a toy during partnership love-making. All that is needed to start is to put some lubricant on the vibrator and apply some with a finger tip to the area of the clitoris, between the vaginal lips and at the opening of the vagina itself. Most women find that at this stage they prefer to use the vibrator without turning it on. Lying quietly on a bed, the door discreetly locked so that there is no anxiety about interruption is a good idea. The very inexperienced may also find it useful to have a small hand mirror so that if need be they can actually see what they are doing.

By rubbing the fingers and the smooth tip of the vibrator gently over the clitoris and over and between the lips there should be a gradual arousal of sexual feeling. This means that extra blood will flow into the tissues in the centre of the clitoris and the lips. Instead of being soft and pale in colour, they become a little swollen, firmer and more pink in colour. Hopefully and certainly after a little practice, the process starts to feel pleasant. Now, very slowly and gently indeed, the tip of the vibrator is pushed into the orifice of the vagina. It helps at this stage for the girl to 'bear down' a little. This technique has the effect of causing temporary but very definite relaxing of the muscles all around the area. Over the course of several days or weeks by practising in this way, preferably twice a day, the orifice of the vagina will, without fail, start yielding and stretching in the manner for which it is designed,.. and without discomfort. When the stage is reached where the woman feels she is ready to put the vibrator in further, it is important that she hold it at the correct angle. The vagina does not go straight up inside like a sort of perpendicular elevator shaft. It is set at a marked angle. Consider the woman lying flat on her back with her legs wide apart and also flat on the bed. In this position the angle of the vagina from its opening is at about 45 degrees (or half a right angle) to the bed itself. That means that it is also at much the same angle to the line of the groove between the legs. So, if the vibrator is pushed straight down towards the bed, not only is it not angled up the vagina, it is pointing straight towards the wall of the rectum which lies next behind the vagina. Angling it too far forwards, that is, more or less parallel with the surface of the bed, pushes it against the very sensitive urinary bladder which is next in front. Pressing against that can be most uncomfortable. Holding the vibrator at the correct angle, well lubricated and when the user is a little excited sexually, the circumstances are just right to try sliding it into the vagina. It should only be pushed as far as is comfortable. Better to try again later and to persevere by small steps than to cause unnecessary pain. After perhaps a couple of weeks or so the girl will be able, easily and with no preliminaries, to slip the vibrator as far in as she wishes. Her vaginal muscles will have become trained to relax and stretch. She will be much better equipped to deal with the first arrival of a real penis. At this stage too she may find that using the vibrator has become a lot of fun.

The use of a vibrator is not restricted to cases of virginity and vaginismus. It is also a pleasurable toy. Not every woman, all the time, has a man available. She may not wish to have one, even. But with a vibrator she can indulge in harmless and enjoyable masturbation as and when she chooses. For many women the use of the fingers to masturbate is sufficient for them. For most, however, unless they are very unadventurous, a vibrator is superior. If for no other reason this may be because, being larger and longer than any finger, it produces a deeper and more enjoyable degree of penetration. There are no hard and fast rules. One of the most important guide-lines in all sexual behaviour, particularly when only you are involved, is to do what you like and don't do what you don't like. But whether it is for pleasure or for the strictest of medical needs, a vibrator may be just the answer. An alternative is the use of a dildo or artificial penis. This is discussed in greater detail in the section on male aids.

**The clitoral aid**

A substantial group of women suffer from a low threshold of sensation in the clitoris. When the stimulation there is inadequate the whole process of initiating a sexual response is impaired.

During intercourse in most of the common positions the penis does not much stimulate the clitoris. In spite of popular opinion to the contrary, when the penis is in the vagina it cannot touch the clitoris at all. The stimulation is produced by the crisp male pubic hair being pushed against the clitoris by the pubic bones. This, together with tugging movements of the clitoral foreskin or prepuce, caused by changes in the relative positions of the male and female organs, produces the pleasurable friction. To increase this friction the clitoral aid is used.

Basically, a clitoral aid is a soft rubber ring which fits around the shaft of the erect penis. Lightly lubricated by a bland cream such as Nivea, it is slipped around the shaft of the penis and about halfway down the organ. Moulded to the upper portion of the ring is a protruding area so positioned as to touch the clitoris on penetration. Penis entry into the vagina brings this area into contact with the woman's most sensitive tissues. Then as penetration increases the ring slides gradually back along the shaft. When fully inserted the penis has the ring around its base and the active area of the ring is being rhythmically squeezed against the clitoral zone.

Several adaptations of the contact area are available but only two are much used. In one instance the area is an inflatable or padded cushion, shaped to compress the clitoris and nearby labia. It is soft and pliable and in this writer's experience is the more widely enjoyed. The other type has a profiled area of quarter-inch long, soft, rubber projections, perhaps twenty or thirty in number. The effect here is more intense, almost a scrubbing effect. Where necessary the profiled area can be continued right around the circumference of the ring to involve both the inner and outer lips, and even to extend back along the perineum and stimulate the anal orifice in the many women who enjoy this sensation.

There is a considerably smaller group of women who feel maximal stimulation not on the clitoris but in the vagina. They are particularly vulnerable as vaginal stimulation is usually harder to achieve than clitoral stimulation. For such patients, a number of different aids are also available.

**Penis rings**

Prominent amongst these is the coronal ring. Like most aids this is made of soft rubber. It fits around the erect penis, not around the base this time but in the groove or sulcus between the glans and the shaft. From the ring a series of soft fronds radiate. These are slender and compress at the slightest touch. During intercourse they stroke up and down against the vaginal mucosa.

**Special condoms**

Problems can arise with sexual aids where couples are still using the condom method of contraception. Many sexual aids are unsuitable for use with these. One example is the coronal ring just mentioned which tends to slip off and is easily lost at the top of the vaginal vault. This is not dangerous as the rings are easy to remove. However, embarrassment may result and some feel they are best avoided. For such cases there are specially manufactured condoms which, instead of the normal very smooth surface, have a variety of stippled or patterned surfaces.

Another version has forward facing projections extending from the tip. These carry sensation up into the vault of the vagina and around the cervix. In many women this area is by no means as completely insensitive as some authorities have believed. Care must be taken in the purchase of these sheaths, as some are inadequate from the contraceptive point of view.

Already mentioned is the question of sexual dissonance, that very common sexual problem induced by the difference in time taken for partners to approach orgasms. Women who need very prolonged foreplay are often thwarted and frustrated. The long period of manual stimulation they need is tiring for their partner, especially if he is, after a while, having difficulty holding back his own orgasm.

In such cases the patient can be issued with a dildo or personal vibrator for use by herself or her partner to initiate excitement and bring it to a level where timing is more evenly matched.

### The dildo

Dildos, or artificial penises, have been known for centuries as masturbatory devices. They can be valuable for women who need a lot of sexual activity or where a partner is for some reason unavailable. Dildos come in a wide variety of shapes, lengths and colours. Essentially, however, they are life-like representations of an erect penis. Usually they are hand-held and operated, but they can be mounted in a light harness for use by a totally impotent male or, in those occasional cases where such an aid is required, in entirely lesbian relationships.

### Vaginal training with Gynatone

A considerable proportion of women seeking sexual medical help are those experiencing a decrease in the strength and tone of their vaginal muscles. A frequent result of the natural ageing process, this is also worsened by earlier pregnancy. A slack vagina causes further problems. Clearly the lack of vaginal 'grip' can reduce sensation and make sexual activity less enjoyable for both partners. Any element of 'sag' of the muscles of the pelvic floor tends to encourage constipation, a feeling of insecurity, and, worst of all, some stress incontinence,.. a socially disastrous tendency to leak urine involuntarily when coughing, sneezing, or during physical activities like games, hurrying upstairs or sex. The repeated urinary leaks feel uncomfortable, ruin clothes and can result in a lingering odour around the sufferer which is noticeable to all. Symptoms can be severe enough to require repair surgery though this is often far from a permanent solution.

It was for the substantial numbers of sufferers from both the sexual and social problems of this pelvic floor sag that various strengthening methods were developed. Eastern women insert hollow spheres containing mobile weights into the vagina where their wobbling stimulation improves muscle tone. (Though one lady using the modern type recently complained that it was too noisy as when she hurried her friends thought her teeth were chattering!) More recently an eminent gynaecologist devised what are called Kegel's Exercises to help re-train the area.

Best of all to date however is a discreet vaginal strengthening and training programme devised by a group of physicians in England. It is discussed in greater detail in a later chapter. Called Gynatone, it is suitable for home use and is easy, hygienic and very effective indeed. (Similar methods have been written up and acclaimed in the British Journal of Obstetrics and Gynaecology. (Oct. 1988, Vol. 95, pp 1049-1053). Gynatone can be recommended not only for those already suffering but for those who, after pregnancy or after their mid-thirties, wish to maintain a high level of vaginal tone, performance and pleasurable sensation. (See Sources List).

### The penis erector

The male is very sensitive to failure. He cannot hide his sexual inability by the simple act of faking that protects the unsuccessful female. So, if a man is going through a period of impotence or just a reduced level of sex drive due to age or fatigue, some words of encouragement, together with a whole-hearted attitude of female co-operation may be all the aid necessary. (It is as well to remember that any man who claims to be doing at sixty what he was at twenty,.. probably wasn't doing much at twenty!)

**The famous *Ring of Confidence***
However, there are many cases where a more positive and more therapeutic approach is indicated and where some form of sexual aid can revolutionise both a man's sex life and, with it, his general health and performance. Pride of place amongst male aids unquestionably goes to the Energising Ring. The modern version of this ring was first devised by a Dr. Blakoe working in Europe during the 1930s. Because of the taboo on sexual matters it was known to very few. Advertising was prohibited. Men went on suffering as they just did not know that help even existed. It was not until the 1960s that men in general began to learn about the ring. Since then thousands upon thousands have been worn with a very high success rate.

Originally the ring consisted of a stout ebonite surround shaped to fit snugly around the root of the penis and scrotum together. A series of small, thermo-couple metal plates embedded in the ring responded to body warmth and produced tiny but detectable galvanic currents. Modern materials and manufacturing methods have much improved the ring which now comes in adjustable sizes and with an unique, simple fastening. The electro-magnetic effect has also been substantially enhanced and is designed to improve circulation to the male hormone(testosterone)-producing tissues. Additionally, the compressing effect of the ring on the blood vessels draining the penis results in more blood being retained in the erect shaft thereby substantially increasing the swollen size of the penis and sustaining its duration of erection.

Use of the ring is by no means restricted to the impotent male. Far from it. The effect of the ring in assisting, maintaining and prolonging erection could be advantageously tried by every man after middle age. The response can be quite dramatic, and most surely no man interested in peak sexual performance should fail to experiment with the effects of the ring on his size, rigidity and durability. (See Sources List).

**Making it bigger**
If the main problem is that the penis is physically too small the only real solution is to undertake a radical penis training and enlarging programme such as Penatone, which is dealt with more extensively in Chapter 16. [See also *'The Lazy Man's Guide to Penis Enlargement'* by Dr.Wellyn Probert MD]. But for those unable to undergo training the smaller penis can have its length or its girth, or both, increased by wearing an extension sheath. This consists of a firm rubber/plastic sheath the sides, tip or both of which are thickened or extended to the required dimensions. Similarly there is available a hollow dildo into which the semi-flaccid or impotent penis can be inserted. When held in position by a light belt, a simulated or assisted penetration is certainly possible.

Also effective we have found, is the penile splint. Although improvements are constantly being made the splint remains a rather primitive-looking device of soft latex. It is nevertheless surprisingly effective. The soft penis fits into the so-called splint which is either self-supporting or fastens around the hips with a light strap. With a co-operative partner this simple device can often enable even a non-erected penis to enter the vagina. When it does, there is a substantial measure of direct, normal contact with the inside of the vagina which is absent when using extension sheaths.

It is often the fact of repeated failure to erect and penetrate that amplifies and prolongs sexual problems. By using one or more of these aids actually to introduce a partially erected or even totally soft penis into the vagina, perhaps for the first time in years, it is frequently possible to break the vicious circle, instil new hope, improve sensation and generate a new and therapeutic confidence in success.

While considering the matter of male impotence, so prevalent world-wide nowadays, mention must be made of the so-called *'Twenty Minute Miracle Method for Men.'* It is beyond the scope of this book to deal with the method in the detail it deserves. Nevertheless, behind this dreadful choice of a title there is what is perhaps the most successful yet simple method of combating impotence ever yet devised. It is a medically developed technique, very easy indeed to carry out and which, the doctors who planned it claim, can positively guarantee that any man with a penis and a partner can have sex including actual vaginal penetration within at most twenty minutes. It is a remarkable claim and, in the experience of the present writer, that claim is one hundred per cent justified. The entire technique along with explanations and the routine for a planned programme is covered most admirably in a book called *'Impotence,.. its Treatment At Home'* by Dr.Richard Silurian MD. The book is strongly recommended to all sufferers and to those who want to be prepared just in case. (See Sources List).

**Help with problems**

This is a suitable spot to mention two other kinds of 'sexual aids.' A few years ago a group of experts in sexual medicine pooled their ideas and produced a short series of 'Sexual Problem Booklets.' There are so far three booklets dealing with the three main disaster areas,.. the treatment of impotence, premature ejaculation, and methods of increasing the low female libido or sex-drive. The booklets contain every up-to-date idea for treatment and cure in the privacy of the patient's own home. They are thoroughly to be recommended.

Another very effective extra in treating sexual problems is to support the general and emotional condition of the sufferer. There is no better way to achieve this than by using hypnotherapy which is a very safe and very successful technique. Several companies manufacture inexpensive, mass-produced, home-use tapes. Those that come from medically controlled and operated companies (for example, *Hypnotone*) are most certainly very successful indeed. Better still though, is to have a tape individually made for you personally. Of course it costs more but is correspondingly more effective,.. and it can be used and re-used for years. The advantage is that other emotional problems can also be assisted at the same time. Into the tape can be introduced methods of combating not only sexual shortcomings but obesity, smoking, drinking, insomnia, anxieties and worries, blushing, under-confidence and so on. Such a tape is an excellent long term investment.

The subject of home- or self-hypnosis is very thoroughly and professionally covered in another book with an unfortunate title,.. *'I Can Make You Happy, - in Just Three Days'*. The book gives not only a full explanation of the techniques of starting and ending hypnosis on oneself or on others but it gives the actual scripts of the exact words that can be used in a variety of problems. It covers things like under-confidence, stammering and over-eating very well indeed, but its strongest success is the thorough and effective way it deals with sexual problems like impotence and female frigidity. It is absolutely essential reading for anyone who wants to get the best out of themselves both sexually and otherwise. (See Sources List).

\* \* \*

# SECTION FOUR:
# THE WOMAN'S PENIS

**Chapter Twelve:** The Past and the Present

Mark Twain, the great nineteenth century author and wit, used to use strong language a lot. His wife thought perhaps the best way she could break him of it was to let him hear how awful it sounded by doing the same herself. Accordingly she began, one day, to use the most remarkable and sulphurous phrases. After a while he patiently drew her aside and explained to her that it wasn't worth her while. "You see, my Dear," he explained, "You know all the words but you just haven't got the tune."

In all too many ways this is how it is with women and sex. They may often lack the sheer enthusiasm and the magic. There is little excuse for this. At long last the few who can be bothered to put down a cheap novel or a hero-biography can read and learn all they need and should know. Sadly, the most fruitful attributes of an open mind and a fertile imagination are too often absent or have been cruelly suppressed. This is largely the result of wrongly taught, incorrectly learned, and tenaciously adhered-to principles. The real differences between men and women are exceedingly few. The concept of the male as a virile, dominant, predatory sexual demon and the female as a placid submissive, frigid nestbuilder is eighty per cent fallacious, conditioned nonsense. People believe it because they always have, because it's easy and because a change involves an effort.

**How big is the difference**

That remarkable medical author Dr.Richard Silurian has dealt with explanations for the differing male and female reproductive programming in far greater and more useful detail in his major book *'Age and Sex'*. Here space curtails things to only a brief mention. In fact the genetic differences between male and female originate from the tiniest of variations. Perhaps only as little as a few molecules out of millions differ. The actual sex hormones are so similar that, as one wit put it, 'the only difference between Romeo and Juliet was a couple of hydrogen and oxygen atoms.' The nerve control of the sex act differs almost not at all.

The thing that is different is behaviour. And behaviour is almost entirely learned. That is, you are not born with it, you acquire it later. There is one inalienable truth. Anything you learn can be unlearned, or, to put it better can be learned over the top of. If your mind is open (and a closed one is just about the world's most worthless commodity), it's a bit like a recording tape. You can always learn (or record) something fresh on it. The capacity of the human brain for learning is astronomical. Even the most highly educated person never uses more than a small percentage of the available learning space. So you can always absorb more ideas, ways and knowledge *if you choose*.

The place where sexual behaviour differs from everything else is that it is one (and the only vitally important one) in which the behaviour pattern is learned other than by watching. Practically every skill we acquire is, for the most part, achieved by the act of watching. Yet, for some totally unexplained and utterly irrational reason, sex has been singled out to be different. The concept that the sex act must be in private, for example, is found to a significant degree only in humans, and by no means in all of them. Although it is now the accepted norm the original idea is built on a falsehood, developed by conditioning and preserved out of a mixture of laziness and pig-headed obstinacy.

There are differences between men and women, obviously. On average men lift bags of potatoes easier. At the moment only women can bear children. There are also a very few sexual differences. For example a man penetrates whereas a woman invites (and that is the word, or should be) a man to enter her body space. It is quite a good idea for the roles to change at least occasionally. A man should be *invited* to enter the space of the anus or the mouth for a change. Even more important, a woman should enter a man's space with her tongue or thumb in his mouth or a finger in his anus. The experiences are worthwhile to both. The whole question of role playing is very important in man/woman relationships. Most roles are conditioned,.. like 'man the ever-ready penis' and 'man the protector' and so on,.. but as they are learned roles, with effort they can be superseded.

**The ultimate difference**

As it is the penis that stands almost separate from a man and actually does the entering of a woman it tends to gain a unique regard. Instead of being his, or temporarily hers, it gets treated like another, third person belonging to neither partner. Really, of course, and especially in the erect state, it belongs to both and should be shared,.. the best things usually are.

When a girl child first notices the penis, her reaction tends to be a mixed one of fascination and regret. She is fascinated by this object she does not possess, there being no obviously equivalent thing that she has and the male doesn't. This brings with it a sense of regret that she doesn't have a penis. Little girls' games amongst themselves commonly contain charades in which a convenient object like a pencil is held in the groin to represent a penis. It is interesting that there is no similar game amongst boys. Men who have had illegal experience of sexual involvement with small girls report that for the most part the girls show no fear or horror of the penis, but rather a marked interest and a considerable willingness to participate. It is only if and when, on rare occasions, they are hurt that an aversion understandably develops. In the large majority of cases little if any damage results to the child. (This includes boys as these too often have sexual advantage of them taken by women). Incestuous relationships, especially between father and daughter, on the other hand, are a much commoner cause of serious mental damage to the child. By far the greater amount of damage usually results from the guilts and fears that arise from the subsequent actions of involved adults if the relationship comes to light. Questioned in later life, women who as children had such happy relationships usually speak with a great measure of warmth about their older partners. Such men, in fact, seldom hurt them. Much of their pleasure being in a kind of gentle revelation and a mutual, sensual exploration which is probably injurious to no-one and indeed may well be beneficial. It is society that is wrong in seeing such relationships as automatically evil, and in responding in an immature manner indicative of personal doubts and guilts when outrage ensues.

**The first taboo**

At an early stage, howsoever, the part of the human body, male or female, which is covered by the pants becomes the subject of restricting taboos. From each generation is passed on the principle that the genitals are private, secret and not to be shown, played with or under any conditions to be proud of. Commonly, many years go by before a girl again sees or feels a penis. By the time she does, it has been built up into a wonder object, a hidden masculine thing. When she encounters it she may be shocked, disgusted, amazed, appalled, intrigued and many other things. She will almost never be indifferent. Commonly it is the furtive hand that finds its way to the excited penis and discovers itself touching the vibrant rod that symbolically has such an aura of masculinity.

Already, at this point, the girl is at something of a crossroads. Every penis she ever meets will, at the first sight or touch, have an effect on her in its way as does every first kiss. But the first penis she seriously handles can mark a turning point. A girl can either start moving slowly towards a sense of pleasure and enjoyment in all things sexual or she can start holding back in accordance with her teaching. An ambivalence will be present in most girls inclining sometimes one way sometimes another. Unless she is emotionally disturbed or too fiercely programmed, no woman will resist her sexual arousal once she has decided that the circumstances are right for her. Hopefully she will find that she can then enjoy sex. If she does, she can become a treasure to her partners and a fulfilled contented human in herself. Alternatively, she may well start the inexorable slide down into accepting the socially imposed role that suppresses her desires and hides the enjoyment and orgasms that might otherwise have been her rightful comfort. It is easy enough to become the woman who expects nothing and gets it. She will make excuses for her clumsy and unskilled lovers, will convince herself that one can't have everything and will come to believe that orgasm is not really important. She will console herself with the incorrect belief that the only joy lies in giving pleasure to her partner. There is immense pleasure in that of course, but there is so much more. The extra, like all extras, doesn't come without an effort.

The widespread propaganda of woman's second class citizen role is so effective that resistance is not only hard but most women never even think of resisting. Until the advent of women's' lib (which did a lot of harm but in all fairness this one morsel of good), a woman who saw the light was likely to be branded as a slut. To be sexually turned on was the equivalent of a life of abandoned promiscuity.

**The modern woman and sexual fulfilment**

To a woman a penis can be pleasure or a burden, a joy or a horror. It can be something to look at, fondle, kiss and enjoy in all its many aspects. Or it can be a cynical, demanding implement imposing its unrewarding will. It can be a fear object or a fetish object. Much depends upon the woman. For so many years women have been conditioned away from the correct attitude that they can now hardly help themselves. (Though it must be pointed out that they have been guilty of blindly continuing the myth into the minds of their own children). Now after years of being talked out of the truth of their own bodies, the onslaught of the alternative view is confusing them. They feel that if they are not sexually aroused and alert at every moment, avidly searching for the bulging trousers and the rigid penis, they are subnormal, sick or at the very least, deprived. The balance is the hard thing to find. The refuge often in extremes.

No sex-crazy woman is really wanted,.. any more than is a sex-crazy man. The image is one thing, the reality quite another. The male literature is full of the fantasy of the lewd nymphomaniac, insatiable and smouldering with lust. Men dream of such women. But I have never yet met a man who having found one (and they are exceedingly rare), wanted to keep her long, or indeed could satisfy her for long either. The very lasciviousness and continuous lechery is a threat to the less renewable man. Occasional lechery is the gift, not the rutting heat of perpetual lust.

On the other hand, if a woman fails to give the penis its due and her sexual potential its head, she spreads a forever kind of misery around her wherever she goes. A sexless woman is without redemption. She neither pleases nor inspires. Her life and the lives of those she can influence become a perpetual mediocrity. Continuous sameness and nothingness are philosophically indistinguishable. If her attitude becomes one of 'I can't do any more than I do' she is declaring that she is too selfish to better herself. If she says 'What more can he want of me' she is guilty of saying, in different words, 'there's a lot I can learn but I'm too idle.' If a she says 'I've done everything I can' it is certain that she hasn't. The person who adheres to a one position, one day, one place sex life and steadfastly declines to encourage either self or partner in anything more should remember that whatever they choose to be missing they have absolutely no right to make anyone else miss too.

After the early stages, when all of sex is new and a bit overpowering, there is no longer any more time or room for unresolved hang-ups. The stand-still personality that really does want the same armchair, the same shirt, the same sex pattern throughout life is entitled to that, but must never obstruct others who are more adventurous. The tearing, burning lust that knows nothing of the tender side of sex is an entitlement too, but one person must never drag another along by the hair.

There is no substitute for a mutual devotion to everything of the giving and the taking that is love. Nothing short of a dedicated and wholehearted involvement in sex will do. Being generous in bed hurts no one and improves the world.

\* \* \*

# Chapter Thirteen: Mutual Techniques

## The female pleasure button

There are three regions where a penis can be involved with creating or amplifying pleasurable, sexual sensations in the female genital region. The first area of stimulation is external and comprises clitoris, its foreskin and the vulval lips. The clitoris is by far the most used of all erogenous zones by the female. The inexperienced male lover will often make a bee-line for the clitoris, or at any rate for roughly where he figures it to be. He has read about it and heard about it, mostly highly imaginative tales of a bulging, throbbing lump he can easily locate. He has been told how it works miracles too, and he is certain that a few quick prods on it will turn the girl into a writhing fleshpot. He should be so lucky! The truth is that the vast majority of women find gentle manipulation or sucking of the clitoris and lips to be the best or at any rate the subtlest kind of stimulation. Less than ten per cent of women insert fingers or other objects actually into the vagina while masturbating. Attention is devoted almost exclusively to the clitoris and lips. Very few indeed fulfil the male misconception that they masturbate with vigorous and violent assaults on their sensitive tissues. Women are no more rough with their genitalia than are men with the penis. Light but busy movements of the massaging fingers are the general rule.

## Inside the vagina

The second area, the vagina, is much less used by women when alone. It mainly comes into its own in the presence of the male. Whereas, as mentioned above, few women involve the vagina in masturbation, the reverse is true when a man is available. Under these circumstances only a small percentage of women normally proceed to orgasm with the penis against the lips and clitoris alone. These are still closely and continuously involved as they are inevitably subjected to frictions and pressures when the penis is moving in the vagina. In and out movements of the shaft alternately tug at and compress the lips and foreskin, thereby stimulating them. At the same time the movements rhythmically squeeze the clitoris against the pubic hair and, behind that, the pubic bone. Simultaneously, this also draws and releases the lips which are attached to its foreskin, thus massaging its sensitive head. At this stage too the deep smoothness of the probing strokes within the barrel of the vagina also contribute. The reception of the male penis into the vagina brings with it different sets of associated emotions. There is a different, more profound sense of union. The act of lying back, supporting the male, clasping him, pulling him close, and opening the thighs to give him access to the inside of the body itself, is a deed not only of physical pleasure but of deep emotional significance and involvement. Penetration clearly also has inseparable associations with insemination. This greatly increased pleasure, seemingly, may thus well be a feature added by nature to encourage progress from foreplay to genital penetration so that the insemination act is not overlooked in favour of available alternatives.

## Beyond the vagina

A third part of the body can also be involved. The inside of the abdominal cavity, which contains so many of the body organs, is lined with a thin, moist, surface membrane called the peritoneum. This covers most organs and lines the walls of the abdomen itself. (It is the tissue that becomes inflamed in the condition known as peritonitis). Opening it surgically causes considerable shock and contributes substantially to operative risk. The peritoneum is very sensitive indeed. To cut it, press it or otherwise stimulate it is to cause immediate sensation which may easily be painful. Sheets of peritoneum cover parts of the uterus and reach down as far as the upper vault of the vagina. Other sheets cover large areas of the adjacent rectum. When the penis penetrates the vagina deeply and suddenly, it can cause rapid pressing or stretching of parts of this peritoneum. This, associated with the swift stretching of muscles not given enough time to relax, can produce unwelcome sensations. Some recipients react with understandable shock and discomfort. Others, however, find it intensely enjoyable and describe an overwhelming sense of pleasurable fullness and fulfilment at the sudden intrusion. Whatever the feelings they are best and easiest produced by a long penis. Small ones can't reach to compete in this particular phenomenon.

Women may also find that the blunt head of the penis can nudge at the ovaries. This may be a good feeling or a painful one,.. every woman has to find out and decide for herself. The woman who enjoys this kind of peritoneal stimulation also often enjoys anal intercourse and, partly, this may be why. Sphincter stretching is usually described as yielding the greatest pleasure from the act. However, the peritoneum around the walls of the rectum can come quite a lot nearer to the anal orifice than it does around the vagina. It is thus more easily reached and stimulated by the penis. To increase the extent of the peritoneal sensation, in either vaginal or anal penetration, two things are needed. First, there must be pre-arrangement by the couple to agree to sudden, full depth insertion without preliminaries. Second the woman 'bears down' (the same movement as in opening the bowels or breaking wind). This has the effect of pushing the pouches of peritoneum as far down towards the searching penis as they will go. It also relaxes the sphincter muscles so that entry can be less obstructed and therefore, swifter. There is clearly an undercurrent of sado-masochistic indulgence in the enjoyment of these sensations.

**Care and treatment of the penis**

After speaking of what the penis can do for the woman, what can she do for it? Treating it with respect is a good start. Masculine, insistent and strong it may be at its best. But if threatened it is disproportionately vulnerable. Above all, it hates unfavourable comparisons or if its owner is in some way humiliated. After a man has failed, been made a cuckold or lost his job, his confidence is likely to be at a low ebb. And in a way it is largely his confidence that inflates his penis. Remember too that the older a penis gets the more it relies on actual physical stimulation. Automatic erection may still be achievable; certainly erotic thoughts, sights and talking can assist matters. But don't be dismayed and above all don't think the partner you've excited for twenty years no longer cares if he doesn't get an erection as soon as you put on your black stockings. You probably need a more careful diet and a bit more eyeshadow than you did. He needs a bit more painstaking stimulation. Growing older is by no means altogether a completely bad thing.

The penis can cause pain. In a tender, unprepared vagina its presence can be both emotionally and physically painful. There is no excuse for emotional pain. If a penis is causing this then either it has no right to be where it is,.. and it should immediately go away,.. or the owner of the place where it is has the wrong attitude. If this is so she should change the attitude or get rid of the penis, - or both.

Emotional hurts apart, physical ones can usually be overcome. First find out the cause of the trouble. The vagina may be infected or may have been injured, say in an earlier pregnancy. A visit to a doctor should be able to put these things right. As for avoiding pain caused by the penis during intercourse, the solution is a combination of preparation, patience, and practice. The virgin or unaccustomed vagina must be prepared by gentle, repeated penetration by lubricated fingers. Patience on the part of the penis means slow insertion with the vagina and penis at the correct angles for smooth movement and after appropriate foreplay to bring arousal to a high level. The higher the readiness the less will be the significance of any associated pain. Subsequent practice will then enable the vagina's owner to concentrate on the good bits, move to positions that reduces uncomfortable bits, and acquire an expertise that reduces discomfort and allows sex to be the joy it should be.

Sex too can be a stage on which a whole lot of other different plays can be acted out. At times it can be where the stresses and strains of other aspects of the relationship are resolved. Sometimes it can be the venue for a display of aggression that acts as a safety valve. It can be a tender, slow, almost motionless merging or a fierce, active, brawling act of animal lust. A good relationship can stand all that and more and can benefit from everything from poetic love to mock rape. [Feeling doubt once about a particular couple's compatibility, I asked them if they had ever considered formal separation. I was reassured by the answer that came simultaneously from both "Separation never, but murder,.. every week!"]

**Artificial pregnancy**
Artificial insemination either by the partner (if he is fertile) or by a donor is now an easy matter. Almost any doctor, given a little experience and the simple equipment, can carry out the procedure. The success rate varies, but efforts can be attempted repeatedly and cheaply. Nowadays, sex is becoming separated from reproduction. Women can enjoy sex and all that goes with it as often or as rarely as they choose, with or without the possibility of pregnancy. There are some positions of the penis during intercourse that increase or decrease the odds against contraception. Most were known in ancient civilisations and remain in wide use today in rural or primitive communities. They should never be relied upon,.. either way.

**Sex without pregnancy**
To avoid pregnancy, the penis can be withdrawn immediately before ejaculation [*coitus interruptus*] thus preventing semen from entering the vagina. (The so-called sin of Onan in the Bible, Onanism, which nowadays is regarded as masturbation, was more probably this technique). Another way is by having the woman on top and kneeling over the penetrating penis. Using this position or by having intercourse with the woman standing, or clinging around her partner's neck with her thighs around his hips, enables semen to drain quickly away from the womb. Post-coital dancing is resorted to by some people. After receiving the partner's ejaculate the woman dances with violent pelvic movements and with the legs wide open, the better to shake out the semen. In western society a more frequent and more successful method is a rapid, post-coital vaginal douche.

**Planting the seed**
Conversely, the wish may be to become pregnant, rather than avoid pregnancy. In this instance the object is to create a pool of semen at the top of the vagina and keep it there as long as possible. One of the best ways is by using the number one or missionary position, woman on her back and man face down on top. After ejaculation the woman remains on her back on the bed with her buttocks supported on a couple of pillows and

with her knees up to her chin thus closing the opening of the vagina and ensuring that the semen stays near the orifice of her womb. During and shortly after female orgasm a reduction of pressure inside her uterus can be recorded. This is probably caused by muscular movements in the uterine wall. The effect is to suck into the womb any fluid lying near its opening. If this is semen the chances of conception are correspondingly increased. So, if after receiving an ejaculation of semen a woman lies on her back and masturbates to [further] orgasm, she may well help by drawing fresh semen up into her womb.

In the woman who has already been pregnant, the opening (the *os*) of her womb tends to be somewhat funnel shaped as a result of stretching. In this instance a good intercourse position for conception is penetration from behind while on her knees. She should kneel with buttocks raised as high as possible,.. a position usually much appreciated by the man too, and with knees widely parted to enable him to get as close as he can. She now arches her back so that she can drop her chest region right down to the level of the bed. The lower her chest and the higher her rump, the sharper incline downwards of her vaginal tube,.. at the end of which is the womb's orifice. Fully inserted, the opening of the head of the penis is pushed tightly against, or indeed even actually nuzzling into, the funnel of the opening. With a little patient practice and with one or other partner also stimulating the clitoris a more or less simultaneous orgasm can be timed. This means that as the penis spurts its semen toward the womb, the womb is in the process of sucking it in. All this improves the odds of pregnancy.

**Cultivating pleasure potential**
To get the best from a penis a girl can do nothing finer than to welcome it and help it. If only women were not so given to silence about sex more men would have listened, and some would have learned. Improvement necessitates learning by experience for which feedback is essential. If a man sees something succeed he'll usually get the message. If he's told about something that turns his woman on, there's precious little chance that he won't make use of it. So, if more girls talked, told, explained, even requested, what they like, they would be sure to improve their man in bed. If they don't they must accept a lot of the blame,.. and they should not complain if someone else does better. (The same implications apply to men too). If, after a year or so of partnership, a penis is just plain boring in bed, then part of the blame is usually hers. A man should always learn what she likes. In different individuals,.. and women must always be treated as the individuals they are, male chauvinism notwithstanding, different zones are sensitive, different positions have more appeal, different approaches please, different fantasies apply and a totally different psyche controls the process in each instance.

There is no limit to the variety of women and to the variety of the things they will like about themselves, their love play and 'their' penis. The essential is to tell. Let the partner watch the way you masturbate. Tell him and explain what you do and why. Let him learn how to please you. Go into detail about everything. Keep no secrets. It is little use saying, simply, 'I like you to enjoy me' or 'Best of all I like it backways.' When you speak to your butcher you don't just tell him you want some meat. He probably knows that. But you tell him what kind, how much, what cut, when you want it, and so on. You give him details and you may well later give him some feedback about what his meat and service was like. It is obviously foolish to give your butcher more detail than your lover. It is out of all proportion to give more detail about your sausages than about your sensual needs. But a lot of people do it.

In the book *'Age and Sex'* which we have mentioned elsewhere (see Sources List), there is a section devoted to Advanced Sex. Although written mainly for the over-forties every word is true too for younger people. The section referred to lists the most used of sensible sexual deviations/variations, how to do them, and how to ensure they are safe and above all, pleasurable. Those interested in making sexual progress could do no better than to study the book. But we mention it here as it is a book that strongly emphasises the importance of what we too have just said. Deliberate and detailed communication between partners is so important to the creation and maintenance of a satisfactory and lasting sex-life that it cannot be overstressed.

* * *

**Chapter Fourteen:** Some Problems and Solutions

A man called Michael Schofield wrote a book on promiscuity. He ran into heavy fire for explaining, quite rightly, that much misery in human relationships is caused by sexual jealousy. Yet this is an emotional result arising from the incorrect idea that a person actually owns and possesses his or her partner. There are plenty of examples of similar behaviour of a simpler level amongst lower animals, for example when a dominant male will keep a group of females for himself by the sheer weight of his power and aggressive ability. Many of our inherited but less desirable animal instincts have been suppressed, or at least modified, in human society. Of all things that might well have been better suppressed, sexual jealousy is one. Yet it has not been adequately suppressed. Indeed it has been exaggerated. There has been deliberately gathered around it a false association with romantic love,.. another very questionable business. Those responsible have had amongst them the poets, the church and nowadays, the mass media. It is a sure sign of higher intellect and logic that some individuals are able virtually to eliminate sexual jealousy from their emotional responses.

**Love v. sex**
There is no rational reason why an intelligent and responsible person *needs* to have his or her enjoyment of sex mixed up with the lofty emotions of love,.. irrespective of what, in fact, love might actually mean to them individually. Nonetheless, we have all been so programmed that we believe the two things to be inseparable. It is also widely held that a man virtually owns his sex partner,.. though he may also love her. A woman, furthermore, must always be faithful. No other penis must enter her, however briefly. She must not really even desire a different man. That is a kind of ownership. Such ownership is to a large extent even recognised by the law,.. though the law's ability to enforce so unsavoury a principle is fast being eroded. Now, there exist plenty of reasons for a responsible attitude towards sexual relationships, even if only for the safeguarding of health and familial responsibilities. However, it must be realised that even these and their desirability are questions of the present and exist within our society only. Not all societies concur. Similarly, not all societies believe that children are the responsibility (or the property) of the parents. For the time being, rightly or wrongly, in our society, we do.

Whatever be the arguments for and against, and there are strong ones either way, the current situation means that there is a severe restriction placed on sexual enjoyment by the cultivated misery phenomenon of jealousy. The result is that most human 'promiscuity' exists only in the mind despite what we read in the popular press. Most humans are promiscuous in their secret thoughts. Remove the exceedingly thin veneer of what we call civilisation or moral fibre, and most people are attracted to quite a number of potential partners. If the restrictions were not present many of the attractions would go on to sexual relationships. No-one would suffer if such behaviour did not cause jealousy. It would be just a question of human nature,.. and human nature is the very reason why, given the chance, most people behave like animals.

**Fantasy power**
Lust, promiscuity and the liberal satisfying of sexual desires then, for the time being, must be carried out largely only in the thinking processes, in the mind and as part of a private dream or fantasy world. Some of those fantasies are astonishing. A demure girl of twenty two who works in a bank and is still a virgin explained to me that in the safety of her own bed every night she imagines she is a rampant sex machine. 'I'll do it with

anyone, Doctor' she said. 'Man, woman, child, dog or the bed knob. And I don't care which bit of me they want to put it in or what terrible things they make me do. I love everything.' That is an actual quote. Another patient, a charming woman of great wit and personality, but who is plain and a congenital cripple with pitifully twisted legs, told me that her fantasies are always about penises. 'I don't care whose they are,' she told me. 'As long as they are huge and fat. I like to imagine them going into me and in and in and in,.. two or three at a time,.. but I don't suppose I'll ever get a real one.' It's a tragedy, of course. Sexually, she is exactly what a lot of men would like, warm, open and ever available, but it is unlikely that anyone will ever find out.

One of the ways of helping women with problems at sex counselling session is by making use of their erotic fantasies. Frequently the cause of their sex problem has been some unpleasant incident earlier in life. This has been the seed that over a period of years has germinated into a full scale disaster. One such example was provided by a woman who saw her doctor quite recently. She was aged twenty-eight and was married with two children. She came for consultation because she had discovered her husband had been having intercourse with her best friend. She had no illusions. She regarded the fault as hers. At the age of fourteen she explained, she had been raped, under horrible circumstances which would have been enough trouble in themselves. She had been molested and mutilated by someone she had known and trusted. She also got pregnant. The entire story was in the newspapers; she appeared in court; she had a difficult pregnancy and a deformed baby that died at two months. The midwife told her she was so 'twisted about inside' (whatever that means) that she would never be able to have normal relations or any more babies for a long time,.. perhaps for ever,.. and that that was often God's punishment for wicked behaviour. Throughout the period she lived in a small village. It is not hard to imagine the talk and the atmosphere that surrounded the episode and the girl in particular during her extended episode of misery. As a result, she claimed, she was sexually quite frigid. She had had no interest in sex from her adolescence on. She had hoped marriage would change all that. It didn't.

Her treatment ran in three separate phases. First it was necessary to go back over the rape episode in the finest detail. Light hypnosis was used as that technique makes it easier for the patient to remember accurately and to discuss more freely such painful episodes from the past. The entire rape was re-lived,.. but this time with adult attitudes and the benefit of hind-sight. It is an interesting fact that the passage of time and the acquisition of the experience that goes with it commonly brings a different interpretation of many unpleasant things. She had held the incident in her mind unchanged in all the horror and detail in which it had originally happened. Dissected and reconsidered in small fragments, in reliable company, and with mature attitudes, the event came to hold a much more balanced, and reduced, importance. In retrospect things are often not by any means as bad as they seemed at the time. She was also assured that she was not to blame for everything and that there would be no lasting harm to her despite people's attitudes and the midwife's nonsense gibberish. Furthermore, she was shown that inside her and everyone else were natural, physical longings which were good and wholesome,.. that she had ideas and fancies deep down that she was now to allow to the surface and admit to herself as they were not only harmless but useful for her future treatment. This gave her a feeling of being involved in her own therapy. Secondly, she underwent a meticulously thorough examination. From this it was possible to re-assure her that all her equipment, her sexual machinery so to speak, was intact, undamaged and completely capable of being used. Now she had a more rational memory of her rape, and the satisfaction of knowing she was normal, and capable of sexual response.

The third part of her treatment was the most important of all. It depended on her erotic fantasies. The need was to find some tiny fragment of natural sexuality. Her instructions were to go home and every day for a week to set aside a quarter of an hour when she could be alone. During this time she would be in her bedroom, completely undressed, and in front of a mirror. As she methodically stroked and massaged every part of her body sometimes with bare hands, sometimes with cream, sometimes with woollen or leather gloves on she would look for places that felt nice. At the same time she would try to let her imagination have full freedom.

I quote the case because it was dramatic. Not all are so. At the end of two weeks she had discovered (not surprisingly) that her clitoris was very sensitive and that she enjoyed playing with it. She found that her thoughts were very exciting when she imagined being raped again. Without going into the psychological explanations, all that was necessary was to see her and her husband together and explain how he could enter the scene. He was very understanding and co-operative, and carried out his instructions patiently until the patient had the first ever orgasm of her adult life,.. when he make-believe raped her in their car on the way home from the cinema!

It was the little foothold that had been found in her fantasy world that provided the foundation on which the successful treatment had been built. It was the miraculous built-in erotic capacity of the clitoris that triumphed. As she came to see, the sole significance of the clitoris, is for pleasure. That is the only reason it is there. The clitoris, that tiny female penis, has no other value than to be the source of pleasurable sexual sensations. It does nothing else. Why then is it there? Why then has nature invented it and made it so exquisitely excitable? It can only be so that sexual pleasure shall result,.. and be enjoyed. Such enjoyment is clearly a naturally evolved, deliberate inclination.

**Group sex**
A woman's sexuality, once revealed, commonly comes as a surprise to her. Many do tend to have a slow rate of arousal,.. though there are plenty of exceptions who turn-on almost at a touch,.. but once aroused, if she lets go of the fetters of her conditioning, she may well be astonished. Examples of this are seen not infrequently in group sex scenes.

Group sex means different things to different people. Here it will be regarded it as any kind of sexual activity where there are more than just two people. Immediately, certain categories arise. A couple may accept a third person, male or female. A man may enjoy seeing his wife taken by another while he just watches, or holds her hand or even takes part and shares her. She may find the situation equally exhilarating. Or she may enjoy the stimulation of the presence of a little competition if she is sharing her man with another woman. Another possibility is of two couples making love individually, each with the usual partner, but in each others company. The erotic effects of seeing, hearing, or just being near another love-making couple can be quite mind-blowing and should certainly not be missed by those who are interested and as long as suitable hygiene and health precautions are observed. Alternatively there is actual partner-swapping,.. this writer does not accept the anti-feminist phrase 'wife-swapping'. Finally there is the larger group sex scene where several people are involved. Again there may be partner sharing as in an orgy or couples may remain together in the midst of the proceedings.

It is especially in such group scenes that women may get their big surprise. It should be clearly understood that most women do not have the wish to be involved in any group sex scenes,.. in advance. They seldom initiate them and usually agree to take part only reluctantly in order to please their menfolk. When the scene is in full swing is when the surprises start to appear. A remarkable proportion of men are dismayed to find that although the idea attracted them very much in the first place, when faced with actually being watched, compared or having their services demanded, they are quite unable to enjoy,.. or even to oblige. The women however may well find the reverse is true. After the initial difficulties of getting started they find themselves at a plateau of arousal that they did not previously dream was possible. They find they are much more renewable than their partners and are frequently capable of a series of orgasms, often with a number of different partners. [One lady patient explained that she had so surprised her husband that he complained to her that he had never known she was multi-orgasmic. Her reply? '*You* didn't know,' she said to him. 'Hell, *I* didn't know.'] A common enough problem arises where a number of incapable or worn-out males drop out of the group leaving a number of aroused yet still unsatisfied women. Lesbian coupling is by no means infrequent under these circumstances. Many women have been rewarded, if a bit amazed, after it is all over, not only at their own sexual appetite and capacity, but at the continuous high level at which they are alluring to men and indeed to other women.

**Nature's basic drive**

Allure is something most women know they have but do not appreciate its degree or its power. Many a time I have heard women state that their partners are oversexed and want to be at them all the time. It is sad to discover that this is a cause for complaint. The fact is that when these 'over-sexed' men are away from home they seldom spend their nights prowling the darkened streets, penis in hand and searching for a likely lay. More often they are in a bar or in their hotel rooms watching TV before an early night. The 'over-sexed' impression they give is because it is the woman who, often unconsciously, is so alluring. It is very difficult, if not impossible, for a man to live closely with a woman he finds attractive without being turned-on by her a lot of the time. He constantly comes in contact with her, has the chance to squeeze a breast or stroke a buttock. He sees her dress and undress. He is affected by her physical nearness in a thousand ways. His instincts are repeatedly being stimulated. Small wonder he gets called over-sexed. Although part of her effect on a man is accidental or at least incidental, a woman must accept a goodly part of the responsibility. For whether she admits it or not, a woman is instinctively motivated by sex much of the time. It is partly because of this that she dresses and preens herself though she might well deny the association. She doesn't put on her eyeshadow so that the girl in the haberdashery will say what nice eye shadow it is. Even the wizened old stick of a spinster librarian who has never seen a human penis, nor ever will, is at a deep down level attempting to attract one when she put on her basic black dress and her row of pearls. The subconscious impulse to be alluring is unquenchable in a woman because it is natural in origin. It is for that reason, though unconscious of the association, that she applies the carmine lipstick that emphasises her mouth as a vivid, alluring replica of a vulva.

There is abundant evidence, as we have commented before, that women and men have a very similar sex drive,.. far more similar that has hitherto been recognised or taught. Women are now undergoing a crash course in emancipation. They are being forced up to a level of freedom that took men centuries to achieve all in the course of a few years. Inevitably this greater rate is bringing a different set of problems. Some imagine that wild promiscuity is the immediate, easy solution. It isn't. Others pretend permissiveness is not happening, try to ignore it, make it go away and remain, themselves, unaltered. Yet others have become quite unbalanced. We have a few shining examples among us today who have become famous as objects of ridicule for their puritanical attempts to be 'clean' and make others 'clean.' The anti-pornographers, obsessed and sublimating. The censorship promoters whose ideas of obscenity are themselves obscene. Priests lauding chastity when they themselves are celibate,.. a perversion at least the equal of homosexuality. These have gathered around them similarly confused and frightened equals in large numbers,.. and then, mistakenly claimed that the existence of such legions of the sadly deprived is the result of good sense which must automatically make their views right. Their dirty-minded campaigns have all the attributes of sick emotions. Such women and even men are seldom able to defend their views with rational thinking. To them the idea is repulsive, of lying affectionately for an hour with a loved one, quietly letting the tensions subside, or gently sucking a thumb or a nipple, or slowly stroking a penis or a lock of hair,.. of sharing a long kiss, each breathing in the breath of the other,.. of tenderly being together and merging in peace and rest before a frantic, exhausting burst of inflamed passion and locked bodies brings the climax of the day and loving sleep in each others arms. Sadly, these activities, which they abhor, are frequently those which they have never actually had,.. or which they have had and lost, thereby growing frustrated and bitter. Either they don't know what they're missing,.. or they know only too well.

**Penis substitute**
In the chapter on sexual aids we mentioned the use to the female of penis substitutes. All kinds of objects have been pressed into service from fruit to door knobs. Even in the Bible a dildo gets a mention. Today's dildos are very realistic,.. looking, feeling and even smelling, just like the real thing. Mechanical dildos and vibrators are the biggest selling of all sex aids. There is even one that goes up and down and side to side at variable speeds altered from a small, hand-held control box. These substitutes have a place for the woman alone, though I find that most are used by couples as a variation or as a fetish object during their joint foreplay. There is no harm in them as long as they are kept clean, and are used no more violently than would be a real penis. The modern cult for using king-size dildos and vibrators two or three inches wide and over a foot long is nothing but a fetish. Kept as play objects there is no harm in them either. More often however, their use has sadistic overtones. Some mildly sadistic aspects to love play are not only common but desirable. Gentle mutual bondage, spanking, and so on all have a proper place in the repertoire. But for anyone to attempt to wield one of these large penis-substitutes and to ram it into the anus, mouth or vagina of partner or self, is a dangerous practice and is to be discouraged strongly.

**Oral sex**
Other questions commonly asked by women concern oral sex. Should it be permitted? Is it abnormal? Is it a perversion? When, where and how often? And so on. Oral sex is not a perversion. In fact in the course of the last two decades it has changed from being

a secret taboo to being a part of most sensible peoples' love play. Oral sex is to be encouraged always and anywhere as long as questions of hygiene are attended to. There is no such thing as too much or too little. It depends on what you like and when.

After the famous Linda Lovelace case at London's Old Bailey (at which case the present writer assisted in the successful defence leading to acquittal), a lot of questions about oral sex were raised. Linda Lovelace in her book explained how, with practice, a woman can take a penis not only into her mouth but well down into her throat. Many will find the technique interesting, some will want to learn it. Certainly men enjoy it. However, during the case and as part of the painfully inadequate case for the prosecution an expert was called to give evidence of how dangerous deep throat oral sex could be. This has raised doubts in many people's minds. Let us now get rid of them. If something, like a morsel of food, 'goes down the wrong way' it goes, instead of down the food tube (the oesophagus or gullet), down the air-tube, (the windpipe or the trachea) by mistake. The trachea is sensitive to unwanted objects and there is much coughing and spluttering until it is cleared. Occasionally large and solid objects have gone down the trachea and got stuck there. That is a dangerous matter. Small quantities of liquids, such as saliva or semen, do not have the same ability to cause a blockage. They get coughed out and present no hazard.

But there is also a weird and wonderful and very rare phenomenon called vagal inhibition. Under the influence of a sudden stimulus to certain parts of the body the throat can close, the breathing and even the heart may stop and death may follow. The vast majority of doctors manage to struggle through an entire professional lifetime without ever seeing such a case. Indeed, if oral sex caused any significant degree of danger in this direction, so common is the practice that every doctor would be seeing dozens of cases regularly. This is simply not the case. If you are sucking a penis you can usually tell from the crescendo of activity when it is coming towards ejaculation. Thus, if you are going to take the semen into your mouth you know when it is coming. You are thus ready for it, can prepare for it, position it and take any precautions you find appropriate. Most ejaculations take place simply into the mouth and onto the tongue. When it is far down the throat the opening of the penis is, in fact, well past the tracheal opening. There is virtually no chance of semen going down the wrong way. If you do have the penis right down your throat beyond the point where your reflexes can help protect you, and if its squirts, and if you didn't know, and if you mistimed the whole business then it just might go down the wrong way. If every possible stroke of bad luck in the world were against you you just might get a vagal inhibition. It is so rare that I have never heard of it happening during oral sex,.. and very seldom anywhere else either. It is virtually a theoretical possibility only especially from oral sex. There is far more chance of getting cancer from smoking cigarettes and far, far more chance of getting run over crossing the road. It is that kind of rare. So go ahead with oral sex, deep-throat if you wish,.. and can, and enjoy as much as you like.

It is not debasing or demeaning in any way for a man to give a woman oral sex. Cunnilingus is a vital and enjoyable part of sex to most normal women. Similarly, it is not in any way wrong for a woman to be a little submissive, to give oral sex to a partner she cares about. Fellatio, or paying lip service as it is sometimes called, is a wonderfully fulfilling thing to give and to receive. Mature minded people are not interested in submission anyway except as part of love-play. It may have a part to play in bondage games which depend on varying submission/suppression roles. But that's all. Oral sex is in no way wrongly submissive or humiliating to anyone. Neither is any other part of sexual indulgence, except perhaps in the mistaken eyes of a confused partner. Mature people want a full, progressive, exciting sex life full of wanton indulgence and free of the unnatural fetters of all artificial restrictive practices. The true humiliation is when a man insults, belittles or ignores his partner, especially in company. That is unforgivable. Oral sex and sexual variety is not.

That people nowadays write and read about sex with increasing freedom is a sign of their growing concern and interest. That sex ideas catch on and get used is a sure sign that a fair proportion of people are getting the message and are starting to enjoy them. But the penis-owner must remember that he has a long way to go and that his partner is often even more handicapped than he is by a long spell of deliberately encouraged confusion. And the vagina-owner must remember and accept that she still needs to be led,.. or that it is smart to let it appear so. It's good for relations.

Female sexuality is not a new discovery. It has always been there. A woman who has abandoned herself to a really skilled lover, even for just one night, may never be the same again. But there is a great cause of confusion lurking here. If a woman has a lover, her affair with him may last for years. But occasional meetings with him mean that the sexual relationship remains primitive. It stays at the level of a new surprise and uncomplicated exploration. It may never make much progress. This simple kind of sex is, to some women, a comfort as it is so undemanding. In no way, though, does it compare with the ongoing, progressing relationship that can be had with a permanent partner. In no way does this kind of sex match up to what sex can really be if both partners give it their wholehearted indulgence. Only this latter is real sex. If you have it you will know what I mean. If you have not, then it's high time to get on with it or you're never going to know.

Few people realise the vast potential of sex yet everyone can benefit from it. The ability it has to relax and to recharge is enormous and continuous. Sex of some kind is everyone's right. Everyone needs it; no one can do as well without. Get some today. An orgasm a day keeps the doctor away, and it's a lot nicer than an apple!

\* \* \*

# SECTION FIVE:
## THE BIG PENIS
**Chapter Fifteen:** Big,.. Why?

If they were to be entirely truthful, almost every man would like to have a bigger penis. It makes no difference how big it is already. Size is something men are very sensitive about. There is a deeply ingrained opinion that big is best,.. that the bigger the penis the greater its ability to satisfy a woman and thus the more pride a man can feel about it. We shall discuss the actual facts shortly, but at this stage one thing emerges. As it is already firmly in men's minds that penis size matters, then it does. No amount of arguing or explaining will change things.

If nothing else in this book reaches and convinces you then let the next two sentences do so. *Men,.. and most women, firmly believe that penis size matters. That alone, is enough to make it certain that penis size does matter!*

Most men have very little idea whether they are big or small. They might have seen the occasional pornographic picture but don't know whether the models are selected for their large proportions,.. which for the most part they are. A man sees other men in the showers perhaps, but since he grew out of the adolescent 'let's see who's got the biggest' games, the normal, heterosexual male will only rarely, if ever, have seen an erect penis. Furthermore, you cannot tell how big the erect penis will be by looking at the soft one. Soft sizes vary very widely even in the same man depending on things like, for example, the surrounding temperature. Once erected the degree of difference from one man to another is much less. Few are less than five inches long and equally few more than about seven inches.

The fear for most men is that that they may not compare favourably with other men. There is a deep sense of competition with other males. This is seen even in cases of being a second husband. Such a husband, deep inside, always fears being compared with his predecessor,.. and it is his penis size and sexual performance which trouble him most about such comparisons. His bank balance and conversational skills are much further down the list of anxieties. If she tells him he is not as good a gardener as her first husband he may scarcely be troubled or interested. But should she suggest that he is not so good in bed or that his penis is in some way less, then that is a very different matter. A tip for her: if you have a second husband,.. or if you have had a lover the first one knows about,.. or even if your partner guesses you slept around a little before you met him, then, if you can possibly do so make a point of comparing your present partner's abilities favourably with the past one. If you can't do it truthfully this might well be the place for a white lie or two,.. or silence. It is a great morale booster to a man to hear his sexual prowess thus compared. It goes without saying that he should make similar comforting comments to his own present partner. Give people a better opinion of themselves and they automatically gain a better opinion of you.

**The advantages of size**

So, accepting that all men want a big penis and that no large proportion of women are by any means indifferent to size, there are two aspects from which the significance of penis size needs to be considered, the real advantages and the imagined. Real advantages are two in number.

First there is the greater ability of the longer penis in some techniques and positions. The actual reach of the penis means that a deeper penetration, to the pleasure of both, is possible when using positions where the disposition of the bodies means that the root of the penis has to be some distance from the vulva. A clear example of this is in vaginal intercourse with him on his back and her also lying on her back on top of him. However far she opens her legs or tips her pelvis down to meet him, the base of the penis is at best two or three inches away from her orifice. A very short penis may be unable to use this position at all satisfactorily. In a nutshell, the longer, bigger penis has the greater potential in every way.

However, it is usually the psychological factors that are the more important. A woman will usually prefer the sight and feel of a good substantial penis. She will feel more influenced by it. She will feel prouder to have its care and attentions. She will have a sensation of pride and achievement that she has been integral in making that penis swell up to its full sexual stature. He, for his part, feels able to show his penis off without chance of ridicule and indeed, with his own feelings of pride. There is no doubt that whatever its actual ability a fine, proud, turgid penis usually wins over a spindly, floppy, small one. To put it succinctly,.. better a good, big one than a good, small one.

Appearance is very important. Beauty, proportion and manliness are factors that succeed. We can illustrate this with a story. If you asked the ladies around a London society dinner table whether (if the choice must be made) they would prefer to go to bed with a black man or a white man, the vast majority would opt for white. Then comes the second question... what if the white man is Ian Paisley and the black man is Sydney Poitier? A lot of women immediately change their minds. It's the good looking ones that win and the ugly ones that lose over and over again. Whatever their talents most of today's stars would never have got their first chance had not their appearance been with them.

The imagined advantages of large penis size in part follow on from this real psychological advantage. It is a natural, if not a logical, sequence of thought that if it looks better and bigger, it will behave better and bigger. Up to a point, indeed this is true. The vast majority of women do find a big penis to be better,.. but,.. they don't always start off with that opinion. Most women, when asked, declare that they do not regard penis size as a relevant factor. But then, most women have, of course, no way of comparing. Despite the so-called Permissive Society many women, even today, will have felt, seen or had intercourse with only two or three penises ever in their entire lives. Women who have had far wider experience give a largely different answer. They still class performance,.. skill, technique, subtlety or whatever appeals to them, as being of foremost importance and equalled only by a courteous and respectful attitude in the partner. But, other things being equal, they like a bigger penis rather than a small one. Many doctors and writers have said otherwise. But their knowledge has been drawn from questioning women the bulk of whom have too little experience on which to have based a useful opinion. A woman's one and only ever lover may have had a smaller penis than her husband but the enthusiasm of a new attraction, the thrill of the clandestine meeting, the desire to copulate, the excitement and the sheer difference of everything including the technique, influence her judgement. She never really compared things on a matter of size alone. So her comments are precious little guide. Women of the world invariably answer that size is most certainly significant. Indeed, professionally speaking, I have come to recognise the answers to questions about the importance of penis size to a woman as a very reliable way indeed of sorting the women out from the girls.

In the ways in which males and females regard penis size there is an interesting anomaly. If you ask a man to choose (if he could) between a longer penis and a thicker one, he will nearly always opt for length. If you ask a woman who has known a large variety of penises for her preference, she will generally opt for thickness. Men do not appear to have thought much about it and length is the obvious choice. The women's choice in most cases is because length contributes less to vaginal sensation than a thick penis causes greater stretching of the sphincter and a greater feeling of being filled. During a medical trial of the Penatone Method of enlarging the penis (detailed in the next chapter) the wives of men undergoing penis enlargement were asked about this matter. Before the trial began the available women, wives and partners of the men taking part, were interviewed. Eighty seven per cent of them were classed as having had little or no sexual experience other than for their present partners. Of these over ninety per cent, when asked, declared that they thought penis size did not matter to them personally though they could understand it mattering to their husbands. Of the remaining thirteen per cent, classed as of wide experience, three quarters confirmed that penis did matter to them. After the trial had been successfully completed and they had had actual experience of their partners' larger organs, almost all agreed that the enlargement had been beneficial to them. They were well aware that the enlarged penises had given them greater pleasure; they also felt the enlargement had increased their husbands' prowess and self-esteem and that these features too were advantageous.

**The well-dressed penis**

There is no doubt that the big penis is a worthwhile goal. But it is not the only way in which sexual advantage has been sought via some way of promoting the organ's ability. Size alone matters but is not enough. Two other methods of improvement also exist and have taken, and still do take, a number of forms. They are forms of adornment and ways of enabling the penis to produce greater sensation. Clearly the first is meant to attract and appeal to the partner psychologically. The second actually aims more to enhance the pleasure of her contact with the penis, it being well appreciated that a sexually satisfied partner is far less likely to couple with another man than one who is sexually frustrated.

Some primitive peoples even today decorate the penis. Usually after any tribal rituals which mark the onset of puberty the penis is made in some way obvious. Examples are becoming scarcer with the relentless surge of civilisation, but amongst aborigines, and particularly amongst the more remote peoples of the South Seas, Borneo, Sarawak and the San Bushmen of south-west Africa are still to be found peoples whose mature men wear stout sheaths over the penis. Customarily these are hollowed out of timber or bamboo which fit over the penis and hang from a cord around the waist. Part of their function is undoubtedly protection in people who wear little other clothing. But to an extent they are also decorative and are consequently finely carved and decorated themselves. Some of the Polynesian tribes who set great store by the art of tattooing beautify the penis with the most elaborate geometrical patterns in a variety of colours. I have also seen, mostly amongst seamen and all too frequently in VD clinics, modern penises which have had the most grotesque designs tattooed on them. The masterpiece was one which was scaled all over like a huge coloured snake and which when erected could be seen to have the snake's head patterned into the very surface of the glans, eyes staring fixedly ahead and with the orifice incorporated as a vicious looking mouth. It was altogether a most formidable looking machine and one which must have subjected its owner to much pain before it was completed. The practice of tattooing the penis, and especially the glans, is mentioned only out of interest, and to condemn it.

Another technique used in some parts of the world is that of embellishing the penis, usually on its shaft, with a series of scars. The wounds are opened without antiseptic precautions, commonly in infancy. They are then deliberately prevented from healing for as long as possible. The result is a pattern of puckering and, to us, disfiguring scars interlaced around the penis. The heaped up and irregular surfaces of the scars are said to be visually attractive. They bring us, however, to the other reason for altering the penis, that of producing additional sensation to the woman. I understand that the women of tribes who so scar the penis find unscarred men less satisfying. This may be just a matter of conditioning; however, I suspect there is a real value. Another example of this procedure is seen in the way that some groups not only open wounds in the foreskin and the skin of the shaft, but then insert tiny fragments of stone before binding the wounds closed over the top. After healing is complete the working end of the penis is a mass of hard projections and irregularities. Its effect on the vagina can well be imagined. Not only are the women easily able to recognise men of the same tribe, but they hold in high esteem the courage of men who undergo this painful operation for the increased pleasure of their womenfolk. There are advantages for the men too, for the women, so accustomed to this extra satisfaction, are far less likely to wander off for a sexual flutter with non-tribe members (so to speak). Quite an inducement to fidelity.

One of the best known and earliest methods of combining attractive penis appearance with performance has always been with penis rings. Sometimes these, such as are used today, are scientifically designed as is, for example, the Energising Ring discussed at some length in the section on sexual aids. To my certain knowledge, however, a different kind of ring can be bought in the Far East; I have seen them in Singapore and Hong Kong. Basically the Oriental Ring comprises a circle often made in ivory or ebony or some finely carved metals. The hole in the centre fits around the penis and the ring is pushed back until it lies against the pubic bone above and the front of the scrotum below. Slightly to one side of its lowest portion is another smaller hole. Through this passes a retaining cord, either a leather thong or a firm silk plaited string. When the ring is in position the thong is passed back alongside the scrotum, up between the buttocks, and around the waist to keep the ring tightly in position. The ring itself has its front surface delicately and deeply carved. During intercourse these decorations rub against the congested and swollen labia of the woman. At the summit of the ring, and often made the focal point of some elegant design, a specially carved knob extends forwards in order to put irresistible pressure on the clitoris. A great degree of artistic expression has been displayed in the making of the rings. It is reported, in fact, that in the late eighteen hundreds when European travellers first began to be accepted in Oriental nobility circles, some noblemen were able to show their visitors substantial collections of such rings. These were designed not only for different visual appeals and for use in different positions, but even to the extent, in some instances, of having the ring or group of rings carved exactly to the measured proportions of the individual wives and concubines, and so catalogued as to ensure the correct selection.

Yet another idea was to remove the eyelids of a goat and after drying, sew them together in a circlet with the eyelashes radiating outwards. This, the so called Goat's Eye was worn in the coronal sulcus behind the glans. Goat's Eyes, now made of synthetic materials, are available in Western countries today. They are examples of a whole range of devices now marketed for the dual purposes of helping sexual problems (see section on Sex Aids) and improving sensation for the female.

There is a tendency amongst Western women, which is curiously yet fortunately absent from their oriental cousins, to regard all these aids as 'mechanical' and to dismiss them, and eschew them accordingly. This view is the exact opposite of the way they avidly welcome any new mechanical gadget into their kitchens. It may be due to some extent to the feeling of shame and dirtiness with which they grew up to believe female sensuality should be regarded. There can be no doubt that it is time attitudes were revised, and that all women everywhere come to see the penis as beautiful, symbolic, and worthy of decoration for the sake of pleasure or beauty or both.

* * *

## Chapter Sixteen: Big,.. How?

If there were a few people who started out reading this book and who were at that time unconvinced about the importance of the penis and its size, there cannot be many left by now who retain the same view. From all that has been said one clear fact emerges,.. and, however it sounds, a fact it is. It is that the penis counts and so does its size,.. a lot. The changing fashions of time have all left man's involvement with, love for, and dedication to his penis unscathed. The penis retains its place at the top of the list of eternally important things. Today as much as ever a man's penis is his most treasured part. The significance of the big penis remains as much a cult and an ideal as at any time in recorded history.

### Penis image

There are only two things a man can do to improve his big penis image if he wishes to. He can actually increase its size. This much desired aim is certainly realistic nowadays. Alternatively, or sometimes additionally, he can create the impression that his penis is big. This latter of course does not convince him. He knows the truth. But it does influence others. Men can be moved to jealousy and women to fascination by a careful cultivation of the image. The drawback is that sooner or later some girl will get to closer acquaintance and may be disappointed and deterred by the discovery that it is less than expected. Hopefully by that time she will be too involved to trouble much. Consequently the process is much used.

The first adjunct to penis size image-making is appropriate clothing. Long, loose jackets and sweaters hide the area too effectively and are counter-productive. Slim-line tailored shirts and short, blouson-style jackets to waist level are better. So are heavy, leather belts with large, spectacular buckles. A fob watch tucked into a pocket in the waistband and having a short strap and pendant decoration hanging over and down towards the genital area is a time-honoured way of drawing attention. Trousers with decorated seams and stitching, or with pockets angled towards the groin have similar eye-focusing results. Some manufacturers have taken things further by using a stout, exposed zip or even cross-over, corded laces,.. the latter also bringing in a bondage/fetishistic factor,.. in place of the more normal trouser closing. Sewing on decorative patches has the same effect. The way in which a man 'dresses' tends to expose or conceal his penis. Trousers being the way they are, a man must 'dress' or allow his penis to hang, one or other side of the centre leg division. If the penis tends to hang to the left (as is commonest in right-handed men from the effects of many years of manipulation and masturbation) it is less obvious in the top of the left trouser leg. Deliberately dressed across to the other side it appears to bulge more prominently, especially if it is away from the thicker area of the seams and bulging against only one thickness of the trouser material.

Underpants too have some appeal. It is true to say that men are almost universally attracted by girls' panties and underwear in general. While this is less true of women, most will find that, if put off by his loose-leg, grey, baggy undershorts, they are less dismayed and even attracted if he wears tightly fitting pants or even a jock strap type of posing pouch. Some girls find an erect penis standing out from one leg of a tight, black slip more appealing than the merely naked man. Whether in pants, trousers or bathing costume, a man has the option of letting the penis hang down or folding it up flat against his abdomen, towards the umbilicus, where it is held by the clothing. Much depends on the clothing itself.

Posture also affects the penis appearance. The tilt of the pelvis forward juts the pubic area into greater prominence. Standing with a slight forward stoop reverses this. Standing with feet apart, knees straight, pelvis forward, shoulders back and the hands on the hips (thumbs behind, fingers in front), or slipped into front (never the hip-exaggerating side-) pockets is an elegant and calculatedly powerful male sexual image posture.

It is also possible to emphasise the penis' appearance by artificial means. For example, wearing an Energising Ring (see Chapter Eleven) maintains the penis with a slight degree of erection and consequent helpful bulging. A similar effect is gained by wearing an erection-maintaining sleeve or even a penis splint which keeps even a soft penis poking slightly forwards. A suspensory bandage works similarly. This is a small elasticated pouch into which the scrotum nestles and having a forward facing hole through which the penis protrudes. It is held in position by light, linen, waist straps. Its chief purpose is to support the penis especially during sporting activities, but it also makes the entire genital bunch stand a little forward of normal. The famous 'Lightsome Belt' is similar and very comfortable to wear with or in place of underpants.

Some men, wishing to go even further, resort to wearing boxes, the genital protecting covers worn over the genitals during risky sports like cricket, wrestling and judo. Putting padding in the underpants is another dodge. It is rumoured that certain well known pop stars whose image is one of intense sexuality have resorted to wearing some artificial objects to increase the appearance of the penis. Skin tight trousers with, inside, a loose, six-inch length of rubber hose is a crude method, but using a penis extension sheath (see the section on Sexual Aids) is more realistic if little more subtle.

It is worth remembering that any or all of these tricks will repel some women; it is as well to recognise that you can't win them all. The consolation is that those who are repelled are, to a large extent, the non-sexually orientated women who are probably a less worthy target to the more predatory males anyway. Other women will be instantly attracted or,.. and make no mistake that it happens, attracted in spite of themselves, almost as if the fascination is too much for them and enough to overwhelm their conditioned reticence. From the chauvinist viewpoint these are the more sought-after and rewarding of quarry.

Methods of increasing penis image are still not exhausted. Technique and talk also help. Making deliberately welcoming and inviting remarks requires a bit of nerve. For this reason it is comparatively unusual and many women will seldom have encountered such an approach. Defensive measures tend to be built on experience and where this has been limited, resistance is often correspondingly low. While dancing he might say something like, "You are having an extraordinary effect on me down there where my control is a bit unreliable." She is at once tossed into a puzzling pool of new thoughts. She may well be intrigued, dismayed, attracted, interested, perhaps alarmed, a little proud and flattered, surprised at his temerity,.. and altogether fascinated. The sudden arrival of so many mixed and unexpected emotions is confusing and can break down social barriers with great speed. She may draw back in feigned horror, she may apologise, she may even deliberately snuggle up closer to have an even greater effect. Either way she is off her guard. He might now say how good the feeling she creates is. Or he might invite more of the same quite openly. Practice is the only way for a man to develop his technique to its best. These pages cannot be used as a foolproof manual. At some point every man is on his own. But everything from "If you're going to do that I'm going to have to wear a crepe bandage/hang a brick on it for restraint" to "If you do that it'll pop out and land up goodness knows where,.. and before you can get your knees together" will work on someone. He just has to try it out and put his failures down to experience. Sometimes actions will speak louder than words. Much-used actions like rubbing the penis against her while dancing are so well known that she is likely to be capable of coping automatically,.. either rejecting or responding as she chooses. Surreptitiously lowering her hand in his for a few nonchalant moments, then, on the turn, brushing her hand lightly or even firmly into his groin is so unexpected that her reaction may be quite different,.. anything from a gasp to a clip on the ear. Again, he has to take the rough with the smooth.

**Yoga and the penis**

In addition to ways of physically or psychologically creating the impression of bigness, men have, throughout time, sought ways of genuinely making the penis bigger. There have been plenty of ideas, potions, balms, magic formulae, and so on. Until recently none of them really had much effect. There is some evidence that a man who has spent years in studying and training his body, for example a yogi, may be able to increase his penis size. Many can raise it from soft to an extreme erection in mere seconds by will power alone,.. then make it go soft again just as easily. But most men have not the time and dedication for these techniques. Substances on the market which purport to have an enlarging effect are totally false. There are some, however, which have as their object the increasing of performance. These range from preparations containing Vitamin E (which makes rats more sexy) to other trash containing mixtures of grease or butter with tiny amounts of pepper. These irritate the penis and encourage it to stay erect. Some forms of medication contain sex hormones, the effect of which is often unpredictable and which in inexperienced hands can be very dangerous indeed. Yet other things are made of reputed aphrodisiac and regenerating chemicals. The effects of most of these, if any, are on the mind rather than on the penis. There are, however, certain very genuine aphrodisiac substances and some of these are very easily available. They are covered thoroughly in other books on the subject (see Sources List), but are beyond the scope of this volume. Rather costly preparations exist like the Regeneresen and Serocytol ranges of products. These are extremely effective for things like general health and the improving of sexual output and capacity. Nevertheless, highly recommended though they are, they have their main effects on performance rather than on penis size. (These and other 'Magical Extras' are covered in Chapter Seventeen).

**Yes,.. it can be made bigger! A proven new method**

It is the present writer's belief, reached after years of study and personal experience, that virtually without exception every normal man in the world wishes his penis were bigger. And it doesn't matter a bit how big it is already. Of course plenty wouldn't admit it or maybe even think much about it. But ask them in all honesty and in private and virtually every man would agree. Those denying it would be kidding.

Women similarly often wish they had bigger breasts, narrower hips or sexier legs. These are all Body Image Problems, or, in other words, dissatisfactions with their personal attributes of those sexual attraction abilities upon which so much of femininity depends. For a man, the very essence of that indefinable thing he calls his Manhood, is concentrated in his penis. And the bigger the penis, the more it pleases him, gives him pride of possession and increases the confidence that satisfies his ego. It is this certainty that lies behind the endless search for ways to make the penis bigger.

Sadly, and as far as we are aware, there is but one method of scientifically proven ability to increase penis size and performance. This is known as the Penatone Programme. As this book is about the penis and especially the large penis, it is as well here to deal in detail with this single effective method of enlargement.

Throughout time men have sought out ways to make the penis larger. All kinds of creams, medicines, magic spells, potions and techniques have been tried. Some worked, most didn't. But the happy truth of the matter is that, medically speaking, many parts of the body can be deliberately made larger. It is a physiological fact that if a part of the body is thoroughly and repeatedly used, that part has a tendency to enlarge. This is what happens when muscles are developed. Used and trained skilfully muscles actually increase in size and ability. This enlargement is called hypertrophy. There is no reason why the penis, or at any rate parts of it and its related structures should not also undergo hypertrophy,.. and they can. It isn't quick but it is easy. To many men it is well worth the effort. It can work for almost everyone to some extent or other.

The first reasonably serious attempt at scientific penis enlargement, the Chartham Method, was invented by Dr.Robert Chartham over thirty years ago. That eminent writer, teacher and counsellor worked in the face of much determined opposition,.. rather as did Dr.Blakoe when he invented his subsequently famous Energising Ring. But words of personal commendation passed from friend to friend, father to son,.. and often, it is said, from woman to woman! Eventually many men who were in the know,.. doctors, wealthy entertainers, politicians, senior executives and the international men-about-town in England, Europe and later the rest of the world, used the method with considerable success. Better however, was to come.

**New ideas for old**

The modern scientific method and by far the best method ever so far invented, is the one devised by several British doctors of medicine and known as Penatone or the '100 Days Penis Training Programme.' In perfecting this method all the various factors of the human anatomy and physiology that could possibly have any influence on penis hypertrophy were studied. Then the doctors and their colleagues sought every idea, past or present, that had been reputed to have a beneficial, penis improving effect. There were drugs, creams, electrical stimulators, stretching machines, herbs, minerals and even magic spells. However foolish they seemed at first sight all were carefully considered and, where possible, tested.

Most ideas were discarded either as worthless or as frankly dangerous. Some were adopted, others adapted. Then the methods that had survived the intensive weeding out process were assembled into a complete programme. A regime putting them all into practice was drawn up and finally, given the name Penatone, it was submitted to the leading medical journals of the day. Most declined to publish on the grounds of injured ethics!

**The method itself**

The Penatone Programme comprises ten distinct phases. There are also a number of 'extras' which can be incorporated into the programme for those wishing to progress even further.

The daily procedure involves raising the local temperature of the area with carefully prepared and positioned warm compresses. This temporarily increases blood flow. A unique massage pattern follows intended to enlarge the penis blood spaces and lead on to permanent increase in dimensions. As the penis is too sensitive an organ for sufficiently prolonged firm massage a penis amplification siphon (PAS) is used to extend the period. The PAS is a cleverly designed vacuum apparatus which reduces the air pressure around the penis and draws blood comfortably into it. It works on the same principle as the way an 'iron lung' reduces pressure on the chest and enables a polio victim to breathe. It is safe, effective and easy to use.

So successful has this approach proved that extensive medical trials were carried out in the USA and the United Kingdom on erection devices using the same principle. Called ErecAid and Pos-T-Vac respectively they are now widely promoted within the medical profession as a first option therapy for impotence sufferers. Both are to be thoroughly recommended. The only disadvantage is that as they are more complicated and have vacuum measuring devices incorporated they retail at far higher prices. (See Sources List). References concerning tests abound including the Journal of Urology, January 1988, and the British Medical Journal, Vol.296, 16.Jan.1988, pp 161-162.

Continuing the daily routine, attention is next paid to the surface of the penis in a gradual process designed to increase its extreme sensitivity to all kinds of sensation. The penis contains countless nerve endings capable of responding to sensation and, like nerves everywhere, their ability can be vastly refined with training.

Finally comes a systematised routine for increasing the size and tone of both the large and small muscles involved in achieving and maintaining erection. This, additionally, further increases available blood supply. Practice periods also incorporate techniques whereby mental exercises which can help erection even without physical stimulation are learned. The value of these in maintaining intercourse for longer periods is immeasurable. Similarly of value are the physical penis training techniques which afford much wider control of the degree of sexual excitement. Keeping this level under control is one of the most effective known ways of combating problems like impotence and premature ejaculation.

**A step further**

For those who propose additional training after completing the Penatone method there is a further stage using a Maxitone device. Maxitone is a siphon similar to the PAS used in Penatone, but larger, stronger and more powerful. It should not be used at the start of penis training, only after successful completion of the earlier stages. Although often sold together with Penatone it is this writer's opinion that the only advantage of this is a financial saving. For a somewhat higher cost those wanting even greater increase in penis size can always buy later if they so decide. The Maxitone must be used with great care but it is a truly superlative instrument confidentially manufactured by a leading European producer of surgical items.

**Conditions and precautions**

For penis training to be its most successful certain conditions must be fulfilled. During the first two or three weeks of the course sufficient time must be devoted. It is also necessary to carry out the regime each day if possible. As with most training programmes in the early stages degrees of improvement are small. If the method is not used regularly these advances are easily lost and results become disappointingly slow. Although small results can often be noticed after perhaps three or four weeks these are usually nothing compared with more final results seen say three quarters of the way through the course. The entire programme lasts for some fifteen weeks and unless there is the intention to persevere right through, the best results cannot be expected.

As well as requirements there are some wise precautions. No man should ever attempt the course while he has any active disease of the genital region. VD, congenital abnormalities, Peyronie's Disease and others (see Chapter 9) could possibly be worsened. The programme is not for such sufferers until medical advice has been sought. Prospective participants must also be fit enough for the more strenuous parts of the regime. It would be wise to discuss this (or any other) course involving physical training with your doctor in advance if you have any degree of heart disease, blood pressure, arthritis or such like. Moist heat from the compresses can also encourage some skin conditions and fungal infections. Water for the compresses should never be used at above warm bath temperature. Massage too can be fairly strenuous. If it is overdone, particularly in the early stages, there can be discomfort and possible bruising. This is most unlikely to be serious but it is better avoided by ensuring a gentle start. Last but by no means least the vacuum devices should never be adapted in any way. Making a PAS work more powerfully is easy but most unwise. It is carefully designed to be just right without any extra help from the user.

**Discussion**

The Penatone Programme is regarded as having reached its optimum after some fifteen weeks,.. whence its other name, *The One Hundred Days Penis Training Programme*. By that time the potential blood spaces have distended throughout the entire anatomy of the penis. The arterial inflow of blood during erection is very rapid and when it is complete the penis is visibly larger. The improved muscle performance from the exercises further enhance its appearance, its angle and its mobility during intercourse.

Acting on the assumptions made in this book that penis size is of utmost importance and, recognising that concern over size is universal and not merely restricted to those of below average proportions, a full medical trial of the Penatone Method was carried out by general practitioners (family physicians) in south-east England in 1975 and again in 1988. All suitable cases presenting were invited to participate. Some categories were excluded for reasons of poor health, unco-operative partners, or men who had previously undergone this or other alleged methods of penis enlargement. Finally, in each trial, sixty four men were selected into two groups, the first to undergo the course, the second to be used for comparison purposes (or controls) only. The length and circumference of each penis was measured each week for the duration of the three months course by a technique devised to eliminate or reduce errors. After that further measurements were taken less frequently over a follow-up period of three months after the course was finished. In the first trial, of the thirty two men who started, thirty completed the course and of these twenty eight underwent distinct enlargement. The actual percentages were:-

| | |
|---|---|
| Number showing enlargement | 87.5 % |
| Average increase in length | 16.96% |
| Average increase in circumference | 15.88% |
| Smallest increase in length recorded | 1.2 cms |

| | |
|---|---|
| Largest increase in length recorded | 3.6 cms |
| Smallest increase in circumference | 1.4 cms |
| Largest increase in circumference | 3.1 cms |

Amongst the controls there was no recorded change in size in any individual. Pages of figures and statistics from the trial were compiled and the entire details were sent for publication to the British Medical Journal, the Lancet, the British Journal of Sexual Medicine and various other professional journals. Again, most declined publication.

The 1988 trial produced overall results differing by just three per cent, thus confirming the validity of the earlier trial.

A number of other incidental features of interest emerged from the trial. For example, of the patients taking part, one hundred per cent, even those who had the largest penises to start, expressed their desire to have an increase in size. Offered, at interview, a choice between increasing their length or their circumference (although, in fact, no such choice really existed), fifty six of the sixty four opted for length. Of thirty nine wives or partners available for discussion, only four said they thought enlargement of 'their' particular penis was worth it. Challenged however with the same non-existent choice between length or circumference, thirty two opted for circumference,.. a very different choice from their men-folk. In spite of these startling opinions, at the end of the trial thirty four wives/partners agreed that the increases in size had, after all, proved advantageous to themselves as well as to their partners.

No significant difference was detected between the results or degrees of success of Penatone on circumcised as opposed to uncircumcised participants. One amusing comment however came from the statistician in charge of collating results. She observed that, considering all the participants together, their overall or 'collective' penis had been lengthened by some three feet and its girth was over two feet further around,.. and that she described as 'a lot of cock!' The discussion on the trial by the independent doctors conducting it left no doubt of their final opinion that the Penatone programme really did work well and for almost everyone.

* * *

# Chapter Seventeen:  The Magical Extras

The present chapter is included at the request of the large number of readers of earlier editions which did not contain it. Although that causes some repetition it is in fact borrowed in its entirety from other publications in this series.

Here we discuss some of the better facilities which now exist, which are nevertheless often unknown, yet which many will find are able to result in vast benefits. As a large proportion of readers are, in fact, very concerned with the sexual aspects of their life and health,... and extremely important they most certainly are, there is a considerable emphasis placed on these sex-related subjects.

\* \* \*

When it comes to life, health, strength and sexual capacity there are a number of additional ideas, techniques and therapies available. Few know about these. They are the tricks used by doctors on themselves and their own families,... though by no means all doctors know much about them or even believe in them, so well kept secrets have some of them proved. Until recent years the only way to get such therapies was by visiting extremely expensive private clinics in Switzerland or the Bahamas. They are seldom if ever advertised to the public. They are the realm of experts and people who are 'in the know.' Most are costly but many are nowadays within the reach of almost everyone. They are the knacks and methods used by the upper echelons of society,... the wealthy, the show business folk, top executives and senior operatives in every walk of life.

Here we call them 'The Magical Extras' for that is what they are. Anyone can manage without them. But if you use them you really will find these extras to be most advantageous,... virtually magical sometimes in the benefits they confer. Try some and see.

\* \* \*

## Regenerative Therapy

The best of all is a form of treatment called Regenerative therapy or RT for short. This is widely used by top people everywhere. Some large companies, well aware of the beneficial effects on their senior staff, offer them courses of RT at company expense. Some even treat the wives too! Every health-conscious person over the age of fifty (and younger still is better), should have a course of RT once a year at least. It is well worth the time and cost.

RT consists of a series of injections (suppositories are also available as an alternative), usually four on any treatment day, and given once a week over a period of four weeks. There is a good deal of flexibility in timing. For the most part the injections are virtually painless and have no unpleasant side-effects. They contain extracts and anti-sera of body cells in concentrated form. The cell extracts are manufactured in Germany under their most stringent pharmaceutical regulations and by the method developed by Professor Dyckerhof of Cologne University. As cells grow, they too become old and less efficient. New cells are created whenever needed by the process of replication,... the existing, older cells literally dividing into two to make two new ones. The cells replicate themselves exactly,... skin cells forming new skin cells, liver cells forming liver cells, and so on. The copying process depends on vital molecules in the cell nuclei called RNA (ribonucleic acid) and DNA. But tiny mistakes do happen. Some of these errors escape correction and, in turn, are copied. Gradually they accumulate from cell generation to generation just as if they were perfect. There is thus a general ageing and decline in cell integrity. RNA can now be extracted from healthy young cells and injected back into the muscles thereby apparently permitting a far more accurate degree of replication to be resumed.

The effects of RT are often astonishing. Some people feel benefit within days though most undergo gradual changes after about six to eight weeks and as new cells 'come on line.' Benefits reported include higher exercise tolerance, better memory and concentration, substantially enhanced sexual performance, better appetite, improved sleep patterns, better skin texture and complexion, increased efficiency at work and a general, all-round improvement in sheer zest for and quality of life. Some say that RT actually extends the life span and this seems likely to be confirmed as research proceeds.

However, whether or not it puts more years in your life, it is already certain that it puts more life in your years! For those few who feel no benefit there is no form of dependency and therefore no need to repeat the courses. There is another hidden advantage. Using, as it does, the body immune system, RT acts, in a way, rather like having a vaccination. When someone has injections against say, tetanus, at the end of a month or two they don't feel any different. No benefit is felt. But the fact remains that they are different. They have benefited. They are now resistant to tetanus. Something similar happens in RT. Even the very few who don't feel any benefit are, in fact, different. Their tissues have been made more responsive, more functional, more efficient and more resistant to the wear and tear of existence. No-one is without these advantages although some may be advantages that cannot be actually felt. Over a long period however RT users are well convinced of the very real benefits. The cost of a treatments varies from as little as about three hundred and fifty pounds (six hundred dollars) for younger and healthy people to nearer five hundred (eight hundred and fifty dollars) for those who are older or less fit to start with.

For those who have no geographical access to injection courses treatments can also be given by the rectal suppository route. Although these are slightly less effective than the injections they are a viable and excellent alternative and should not be missed by those living overseas and who cannot therefore attend in person.

WARNING: There are self-styled clinics in London and elsewhere offering these and similar courses at extortionate prices. Some are headed by medically non-qualified quacks and con-men who do not hesitate to exploit the old, the sick and the frightened with worthless substitute programmes for huge fees. Some even employ qualified doctors and pay them handsomely to act as 'respectable' front-men. It is a deplorable practice and should be forbidden by law. When you go for RT be certain you are treated by a properly qualified physician and, if you are charged more than five hundred pounds ($750), suspect that you are being cheated. (See Sources List).

For the sexually conscious there are two specialised forms of RT that can be used to concentrate particularly on the sexual system tissues. As they too are in suppository form and of narrower, specific target zones, they are far less costly than ordinary, full therapeutic courses. Costs are also kept down as demand ensures that they can be manufactured in far larger and more economical quantities. There are several varieties available, the best being known as Masculone and Feminone, as their names suggest, designed for men and for women respectively. These suppositories are of high quality, being manufactured in Switzerland under the well-known, scrupulously precise supervision of the pharmaceutical department of the Swiss Government Health Authority.

Masculone contains tissue-specific antisera from the entire range of male sexual tissues,.. testicle, erectile tissue, nerve supply tissue, spinal cord and so on. Feminone is similar but of course contains ovary antisera in place of testicular. A full course is about thirty suppositories, one every second or third night. The failure rate,.. and every medical treatment does have a failure rate,.. is very low, almost everyone feeling at least some degree of benefit. This is usually noticed starting within the first two weeks. However these preparations are only designed and expected to work on those whose sexuality is below par. Nothing will raise the sexual level of output and performance above what is the proper maximum in their given circumstances. It is fair to say, in view of this, that virtually everyone will benefit who needs to. Conversely, those who do not benefit, do not because they are already at peak. At worst then these suppositories afford an excellent test of sexuality.

They either do you a lot of good, or, if they don't appear to help they have at least shown you that you are pretty good anyway. For this reason the present writer suggests a first investment in only ten suppositories and the rest of the course to follow providing that the new user is amongst the successful ones. (See Sources List).

**Female problems**

There is also a common female problem which might well need attention and which, in affected couples, can be most successfully treated at the same time. This is the matter of the 'weak pelvic floor' and its consequences. If you were able to look at a human skeleton you would notice that the pelvis is in fact a kind of bowl made of bones. But the bowl has no bottom! Anything you put in it would fall straight through. In the living body the bottom of the bowl consists of several complex sheets of muscle, tough, and elastic in consistency, which stretch across the 'missing' areas and seal them. In the female these sheets of muscle are perforated by the three body openings, the urethra to void urine, the rectum to void faeces and the vagina for sexual-reproductive purposes.

As a woman ages, or if she becomes overweight, if she suffers from constipation, and if she has gone through the pressures of childbirth once or twice, it is very likely that the straining involved will have weakened the muscle sheets. When they lose elasticity there arises the condition known as pelvic floor sag. The uterus, the bladder and sometimes the rectum too droop down lower in the pelvis to the extent that the cervix of the womb may even appear at the vaginal orifice.

This has a number of considerable inconveniences. Sudden physical efforts, running upstairs, coughing and sneezing cause the leakage of small quantities of urine. Tennis is out of the question. The constant soiling of clothing and the associated odours make social contacts very embarrassing. Sexually the vagina loses its grip and the slack orifice is correspondingly affords only reduced sensation levels to its owner The partner too quickly misses the delight of pressure on his entering penis. If the uterus has sagged down he cannot enter anyway as the vaginal space is already filled by the displaced uterus. The overall decrease in sexual pleasure comes at a time in life when such limitations are notably counter-productive. Statistics suggest at least one woman in six suffers at some stage of life or other,.. mostly in silence as only one in ten of those goes to her doctor about it.

There are a number of methods of treating pelvic floor sag. The commonest is the insertion of a ring or pessary. This is pushed up the vagina then braced fore and aft between the spine and the pubic bone, thereby propping up the drooping organs. It is a generally successful method. But it does mean frequent removals for cleaning and to adjust size as time goes by. As with any foreign body there is a tendency to infection in the vagina and commonly an unpleasant smelling discharge of pus and vaginal debris troubles the patient and those of her associates within smelling range. Under these conditions, sex appears to become less desirable

Surgical repair or colporrhaphy is the ultimate medical solution. In this the sagging muscles are exposed and dissected out, drawn together firmly and stitched into their new positions. Although not a dangerous operation the discomfort of surgery in this tender zone can be well imagined. Nevertheless results are generally good though recurrence is common.

Before resorting to either pessaries or surgery, there is now a far superior first line of defence. The cause of the problem is weak muscles. Of all parts of the body muscles are amongst the easiest and most successful to train so why not re-train the muscles to do their own job properly again? This is the sound argument that has resulted in the development of such concepts as Kegel exercises, Faradism and the new Gynatone methods of therapy. Re-training has proved to be successful in up to 40% of cases. It saves surgery, sex lives and happy marriages.

Decades ago Kegel introduced his exercise programme for the pelvic muscles. His method was simple but moderately effective. However, being proposed at a time when discussion of sexual matters was frowned upon and most ladies ignored rather than sought treatment for 'trouble down below' the idea never caught on. Faradism has had similar, undeserved lack of wide acceptance. It involves electrical muscle stimulation through the perineal area, the resulting contractions being intended to re-train the weak tissues.

In recent years a new concept has been developed. The same group of doctors who developed Penatone and other devices, got together to devise a home treatment for pelvic floor sag. They collected every known idea then tested them rigorously. Many were discarded others adopted. Eventually the useful methods that had passed all the tests were assembled into an overall programme that was inexpensive and could be used by the woman in the privacy of her own home and without visits to doctors or the need for outside help. This is the Gynatone Programme, which has since had the approval not only of doctors and gynaecologists but of many, many users world wide. It has also been extensively reported in medical journals. It should certainly be tried by sufferers before they opt for other more heroic and costly methods. An alternative to the use of Gynatone is training with a series of insertable vaginal weight cones. Suppliers will be found in the Sources List.

**Aphrodisiacs**

Aphrodisiacs are declared by some to be non-existent. They are fondly believed to exist by many others. The fact is that aphrodisiacs do exist in that there are things which improve human sexual arousal, response, staying power, performance and pleasure.

Detailed discussion is beyond the scope of this book and is far better covered elsewhere (See Bibliography List).

The unfortunate thing is that many aphrodisiacs and substances have side-effects that are dangerous in doses that are likely to have any effect. Spanish Fly (cantharides) is so dangerous that there are liable to be criminal charges in the event of mishap. Gold and silver salts, so popular with Asiatic populations, can cause heavy metal poisoning if only from the toxic contaminants like lead and tin that they frequently contain. Ginseng can cause insomnia, diarrhoea and blood pressure. Alcohol works in small doses as probably do Pethidine and Strychnine though poisoning by these is too likely to justify the risk.

Some foods are known to have aphrodisiac qualities as have some herbal decoctions. A new technique is currently being developed and holds out perhaps the greatest possible hope. A panel of doctors, pharmacists, herbalists and homoeopaths recently pooled their knowledge and experience. After scouring the extensive literature they selected the most successful known ingredients. These herbal remedies have been subjected to extraction and potentisation radionically and are now under test as homoeopathic drops taken under the tongue or in small tablets. It is expected that they will combine efficiency as an aphrodisiac for men and women with the well known safety record of homoeopathic and herbal medicines. If they become commercially available it is intended to mention them in later editions.

**Hypnotherapy and self-hypnosis with home tapes**

Of all methods available for training and improving the mind, which is a vital component of mastering so many sexual shortcomings, hypnosis is by far the best. It is also the most fun. And furthermore, whatever the main reason it is used, for example in impotence therapy, it has huge advantages spilling over into other areas as a bonus. It is a technique that offers a whole series of benefits in just one small, easy package.

It is worth getting a few things straight. Hypnosis is not the way it usually appears in movies. It is not necessary for someone to wave hands or shining diamond rings in front of your eyes. At no time are you subjected to the will or command of the therapist. At no time is your own will-power lost. At no time can you be made to do something which is against your political, religious or moral convictions.

Many of the things which make us unhappy can be improved by hypnosis. As unhappiness states are counter-productive in any sexuality programme, this can only be for personal benefit. Hypnosis can combat numerous kinds of anxieties, phobias and damaging habits. Anxiety over examinations, interviews or a new job, over public speaking or a forthcoming marriage, can all be helped. So can psychological phobias such as those of spiders, flying, enclosed spaces, heights and so on. Emotional problems like underconfidence, blushing, stammering, will also nearly always respond. Hypnosis should also be used for a variety of self-destructive habits like heavy smoking, heavy drinking, and over-eating; these can usually be much improved or stopped altogether by hypnosis.

So can most sexual problems,... which is why the subject is dealt with here in such detail. And its value does not end there. For hypnosis is also immensely valuable in enhancing the sexual performance of a perfectly normal, healthy sexuality too. (For even greater help in methods of using self-hypnosis in a variety of ways, see books and manuals on Home Hypnosis in the Sources List).

While most people find it easier to learn hypnosis from an already-trained hypnotherapist, funds are not always available. Even so, money is well spent on learning the techniques of self-hypnosis also known as self- or auto-hypnosis. You can learn it yourself from a tape very efficiently, for example by using such excellent systems as Hypnotone cassettes,.. and for many different purposes. If you have the kind of mind you think could be expanded and trained,.. and most can, then do not be without the benefits of self-hypnosis. It is easier than you think, by far.

\* \* \*

**The Final Conclusion**

So, the penis matters,.. and the big penis matters too. The heart and soul of both man and woman is gladdened by this splendid, power-bearing and pleasure-bestowing arm of flesh. The man who has read this book will have gained much knowledge about it. He will know what his penis is, how it grows, how it is built and how it works. He will know of the importance of his penis in the worlds of art and literature. He can put to good use his new understanding of penis techniques, the exploitation of its sexual prowess and the curing of its faults. He knows how to project its image. He knows of things like rings and training and enlarging programmes that can make it bigger and better than ever before. And he knows of those magical extras that can improve his sex life and add to the duration of his performance.

But he must remember that if he has a big penis, gradually it will become known,.. especially if he brags about it, or if others do,.. and ladies are notoriously prone to brag of such things amongst each other. Once it becomes generally known then the time will surely come when some other jealous man will complain to his partner that that particular man ".. ought to be bloody well hung."

With luck, and under her breath, that partner might just be able to reply, "Oh he is, my Dear,.. he really, *really* is!"

\* \* \*

# APPENDIX
## SOURCES LISTS and BIBLIOGRAPHY:
Bibliography:
[Books, Booklets, Folios, Manuals and Tapes by staff of the Kent Private Clinic]
**Books:**

**AGE & SEX:** by Dr.Richard Silurian MD: Amongst other remarkable and little known secrets this book explains an astonishing range of sexual techniques, variations and deviations that can treble the sexual repertoire for Advanced Lovers. (*)

**IMPOTENCE:** by Dr.Richard Silurian MD: A full length and detailed description of causes and cures including *The Twenty Minute Miracle Method for Men!* This technique alone guarantees vaginal penetration within minutes. (*)

**THE PENIS:** by Dr.Dick Richards MD: Probably the most detailed booklet ever for non-professionals on this subject. This tenth edition, tells everything about how to enlarge the penis as well as its training and the developing of performance in every way.
(*)

**APHRODISIACS:** by Dr.Steven Roles MD: How to find and safely use simple, astonishingly effective aphrodisiacs to improve your sex life. It is far easier than you've been told,... and they really *DO* exist! (*)

**HOME-HYPNOSIS:** by Dr.Richard Silurian MD: Using easy hypnosis techniques on self and others can help produce fabulous sex. This book gives *actual scripts* to be used in a wide series of possible situations. Also covers weight loss, confidence boosting, quitting smoking and several other useful procedures. (*)

**THE LAZY MAN'S GUIDE TO PENIS ENLARGEMENT:** by Dr.Wellyn Probert MD. A no-nonsense book devoted entirely to the why, where, how and how much of penis enlargement. (*)

**THE GOOD NEWS ABOUT CANCER:** by F.Hourigan and Dr.B.Richards. A remarkable book. The authors have researched earlier, since forgotten but very successful methods of cancer therapy. They have integrated them with modern orthodox and 'alternative' methods, to form the world's first easy-to-follow routine for home or self-therapy even in places where no medical help exists. They promise a 90% success rate.
*"Someone YOU know needs this book."*

**IRRITABLE BOWEL SYNDROME:** by Dr.Hugh Cross MD. Perhaps the clearest, easiest and simplest book on the market anywhere that shows how to prevent, diagnose and treat [at home] this common and most embarrassing condition. Two million people suffer in UK alone,.. most of them needlessly.

**PSYCHIC COMMAND [& PSYCHIC SEXUAL COMMAND]** by Dr.Bryan d'Gwent MD. Perhaps the most remarkable book you will ever read. Shows how to master the previously secret, un-published techniques of Psychic Command which enable one person to command and influence others by remote control and absolutely without them knowing. Use it to improve friendships, business relationships,.. and sexual advances,.. secretly. Astonishing. (*)

*'A life-changing book. If only I'd known of it years ago!'* [Prof.Patrick Dawkins]

**Folios:** (*)

Ten Erotic Short Stories for Ladies: two folios with line illustrations of the stories as recorded on the audiocassette below. Absolutely no rude words and no pornography. This is *EROT*ography at its finest,.. sensual, instructive, exciting,... certainly not for the faint-hearted.

**Audio-cassette:** (*)

**Ten Erotic Short Stories for Ladies.** Bedroom listening? For gentlemen too! (On two cassettes)

**Video-cassette:** (*)

**'IMPOTENT?... You Don't Have To Be.'** The first explanatory video that, in total privacy, shows you the causes of your problem, how to diagnose it and treat it with all the methods now available. Pays special attention to the Twenty Minute Miracle Method which *guarantees* vaginal penetration in minutes! Also shows techniques of how to use Energising Rings and Penis Enlargement. [Sexually illustrated and explicit. Not for sale to minors].

**Booklets and Manuals:**

Sexual Problem Series: (*)

1. Erectile Inedequacy.(Impotence)
2. Increasing Female Libido.(Frigidity)
3. Premature Ejaculation.

(*) All available from:

DASH Publishing
P.O.Box 22
Plymstock, Plymouth PL9 0YU
England
Phone: 01752-481717
Fax: 01752-480707
E-Mail: dash-publishing@dept-o.demon.co.uk

\* \* \*

**Sources:**

For the convenience of readers, full details, current prices and supplies concerning the books mentioned in the above text and the following products can now all be obtained through the central address above, [DASH Publications], the mail-order distributor for the Kent Private Clinic:

Energising Rings (Blakoe)
GYNATONE, Pelvic Floor Programme
MASCULONE and FEMINONE, Sexual Anti-Sera Suppositories
PENATONE Penis Training and Enlarging Programme
ERECTONE, erection cream
SEX MAGNETRODE

*Regenerative Therapy:* For all data and details on full and booster courses write in confidence to The Senior Consultant, Kent Private Clinic, [as below].

*Hypnotherapy* and Personal Audio-Cassettes and
Hypnotherapy Course for home-study and learning [Supervised].

                Kent Private Clinic
                Sandwich, Kent. England. CT13 9DL

*Postal Advice:*    **Lady Charles' Advisory Bureau**
                PO.Box 75
                Sandwich CT13 9RT
                England

                           \* \* \*

To obtain further information on any book or item and in complete confidence, please cut out and mail this page:

[No obligation incurred]

## THE PENIS    DR. DICK RICHARDS MD

From:
Your name and address here please

Name: ........................................................................................
Address: ....................................................................................

............................................................................

..................Post/Zip code ...........................

To:
DASH Publishing
PO Box 22
Plymstock,
Plymouth PL9 0YU
England

Phone: 01752-481717
Fax: 01752-480707

Dear Sirs,
Yes please,.. I'd like to receive further information entirely free and confidentially. Please rush it to me at the above address.
I certify that I am above eighteen years of age.

Signed
..............................................................

DASH Publishing
PO Box 22
Plymstock,
Plymouth PL9 0YU
England

Stamp required